GW01551370

CASE STUDIES
FROM
CHINESE ACUPUNCTURE EXPERTS

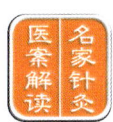

Project Editors: Huang Lei, Shen Cheng-ling & Liu Shui
Book Designer: Li Xi
Cover Designer: Li Xi
Typesetter: Wei Hong-bo

CASE STUDIES
FROM
CHINESE ACUPUNCTURE EXPERTS

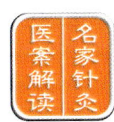

Wang Hong-cai, Ph.D. TCM
Professor of Chinese Medicine
Zheng Zhen-zhen, M.S. TCM
Wang Hui-zhu
Professor of Chinese Medicine

Institute of Acupuncture and Moxibustion, China Academy of Chinese Medical Sciences
China Beijing International Acupuncture Training Centre
World Health Organization Collaborating Centre for Traditional Medicine

Edited by
Michael Max, L.Ac

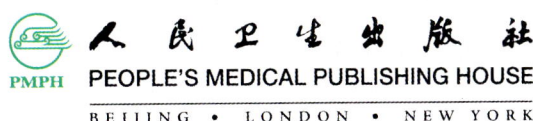

人 民 卫 生 出 版 社
PEOPLE'S MEDICAL PUBLISHING HOUSE
BEIJING • LONDON • NEW YORK

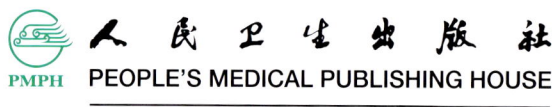

人民卫生出版社

PEOPLE'S MEDICAL PUBLISHING HOUSE

BEIJING • LONDON • NEW YORK

Website: http://www.pmph.com

Book Title: **Case Studies from Chinese Acupuncture Experts**
名家针灸医案解读

Contact address: Bldg 3, 3 Qu, Fangqunyuan, Fangzhuang, Beijing 100078, P.R. China, phone/fax: 8610 6769 1034, E-mail: pmph@pmph.com

For text and trade sales, as well as review copy enquiries, please contact PMPH at pmphsales@gmail.com

---

Disclaimer

This book is for educational and reference purposes only. In view of the possibility of human error or changes in medical science, neither the author, editor, publisher, nor any other party who has been involved in the preparation or publication of this work guarantees that the information contained herein is in every respect accurate or complete. The medicinal therapy and treatment techniques presented in this book are provided for the purpose of reference only. If readers wish to attempt any of the techniques or utilize any of the medicinal therapies contained in this book, the publisher assumes no responsibility for any such actions.

It is the responsibility of the readers to understand and adhere to local laws and regulations concerning the practice of these techniques and methods. The authors, editors, and publishers disclaim all responsibility for any liability, loss, injury, or damage incurred as a consequence, directly or indirectly, of the use and application of any of the contents of this book.

First published: 2009
ISBN: 978-7-117-11808-8/R · 11809

Cataloguing in Publication Data:
A catalogue record for this book is available from the
CIP-Database China.

Printed in The People's Republic of China

ISBN 978-7-117-11808-8

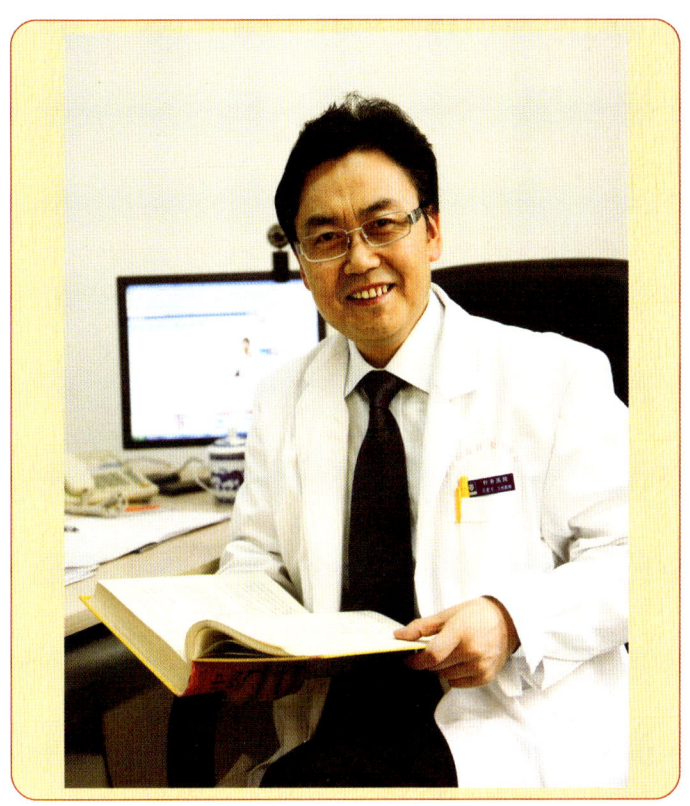

Wang Hong-cai, a professor of the China Academy of Chinese Medical Sciences, doctor of medicine, doctoral advisor, and assistant director of the China Beijing International Acupuncture Training Centre of the World Health Organization Collaborating Centre for Traditional Medicine (Acupuncture). He was a student of Cheng Xin-nong, Guo Cheng-jie, and Zhu Li-xia.

Invited to more than 30 countries for academic exchanges and administering treatments, he served the Ministry of Foreign Affairs and State Administration of Traditional Chinese Medicine, and has treated international leaders, including the president of India and the leaders from Iraq and Indonesia. He was the former deputy secretary-general of the World Federation of Acupuncture-Moxibustion Societies.

Preface

Acupuncture and moxibustion are arts that embody the unique wisdom of the Chinese people. It has found its way into other cultures and in more than 140 countries it has taken root and developed rapidly; In order to allow more people to understand and use it well, a systematic study of medical records of well-known contemporary experts is presented here to demonstrate its clinical effectiveness.

These 150 medical records, covering 70 diseases, have been carefully selected. Each case explores both a unique disease pattern and gives a generalized overview of the disease. In this book, great importance is attached to the particular treatment methods these expert practitioners use in approaching different illnesses. For example, there is Professor Guo Cheng-jie's treatment of mammary diseases and Professor Shao Jing-ming's methods of treating asthma. Special attention is paid to different treatment styles for the same disease; in this way you can see the various ways that can yield results.

Case Studies from Chinese Acupuncture Experts was written at the request of foreign doctors and used as a reference book for teaching acupuncture. We would be greatly delighted if it benefits our readers. Your suggestions and comments are highly appreciated.

Special thanks should be given to Prof. Cheng Xin-nong, of the China Academy of Engineering, for his great support and guidance in compiling this book. Gratitude also to Dr. Walter Liu, MHA, M. D., Grace Shen, Ph. D. TCM, and May H. Rao, M.S .TCM, of the People's Medical Publishing House for their great help in planning and publishing of this book.

Finally, we sincerely hope that more and more foreign friends will come to understand acupuncture and Chinese culture through the study of this book.

One world, one dream. Hand in hand, for tomorrow.

Wang Hong-cai
Eve of the Beijing Olympic Games

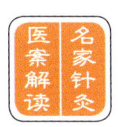

TABLE OF CONTENTS

CHAPTER 1: INTERNAL DISEASES

CHAPTER 2: GYNECOLOGICAL AND PEDIATRIC DISEASES

IX

CHAPTER 3: DISEASES OF EYES, EARS, NOSE AND THROAT

CHAPTER 4: SKIN DISEASES, EXTERNAL DISEASES

CHAPTER 5: OTHERS

CHAPTER 1 INTERNAL DISEASES

Internal Diseases

Gynecological and Pediatric Diseases

Diseases of Eyes, Ears, Nose and Throat

Skin Diseases, External Diseases

Others

COMMON COLD

Yang Jie-bin's Medical Record

Yang, male, 35, first visit was on April 28, 1976

【Chief Complaint】
Headache and fever for one day

【Present Medical History】
The patient had slept without covering himself to stay warm, and on the following day began to experience dizziness, headache, aversion to wind cold without sweating which then turned into a fever, along with a runny nose, itchy throat, cough, insipid taste in the mouth, but with normal urine and stools.

【Examination】
Body temperature 40℃ (104℉), white moist tongue coating, with a floating and tight pulse

【Diagnosis】
Common cold (wind cold constraining the exterior)

【Treatment Principles】
Dispel wind cold, resolve the exterior by means of diaphoresis

【Treatment】

DU 14 (*dà zhuī*)   BL 12 (*fēng mén*)   *tài yáng* (EX-HN5)

LI 4 (*hé gǔ*)

Moxibustion was applied after needling DU 14 (*dà zhuī*). Cupping was applied after needling BL 12 (*fēng mén*). *Tài yáng* (EX-HN5) and LI 4 (*hé gǔ*) were punctured with reducing method. After one treatment, he sweated and his fever relieved. After two treatments, his symptoms were greatly reduced. After three treatments, he was cured.

【Note】

　　Tài yáng (EX-HN5) and LI 4 (*hé gǔ*) were reduced to relieve exterior symptoms by dispelling wind through sweating. BL 12 (*fēng mén*) was punctured and cupped to dispel wind and diffuse the lung to relieve exterior symptoms. DU 14 (*dà zhuī*), the intersecting point of all yang channels, was punctured to strengthen the exterior and then treated with moxibustion to dispel cold. A course of three acupuncture and moxibustion treatments cured the patient.

Cheng Xin-nong's Medical Record

　　Liu, male, 33, first visit was on September 6, 1986

【Chief Complaint】

　　Fever, cough, headache, neckache and backache for 10 days

【Present Medical History】

　　Patient was attacked by cold while sleeping at night 10 days previously. On the following morning he woke with a fever and coughing. He took *Sù Xiào Gǎn Mào Jiāo Náng* (Quick Effect Common Cold Capsule, 速效感冒胶囊) and *Bǎn Lán Gēn Chōng Jì* (Radix Isatidis Infusion, 板蓝根冲剂) but it did not relieve his symptoms. After taking the herbs his back felt cold, with a headache concentrated in the occipital region, soreness in the neck and back, and his entire body was achy. He had coughing with a sore throat, and profuse thin yellow sputum, a lack of taste, and slept poorly. His urine was dark yellow; stools were normal.

【Examination】

　　Tongue borders and tip were red, with a thin white dry coat, the pulse was floating and rapid

【Diagnosis】

　　Common cold (due to cold in the exterior, with interior heat)

【Treatment Principles】

Dispel wind cold, promote diffusion of the lung to disperse heat

【Treatment】

DU 14 (*dà zhuī*)	GB 20 (*fēng chí*)	BL 13 (*fèi shù*)
BL 9 (*yù zhěn*)	LI 17 (*tiān dǐng*)	*tài yáng* (EX-HN5)
BL 2 (*cuán zhú*)	LU 7 (*liè quē*)	LI 4 (*hé gǔ*)
LU 11 (*shào shāng*)		

LU 11 (*shào shāng*) was bled using a three-edged needle. Other points were punctured with filiform needles that were retained for 30 minutes. After three treatments the symptoms disappeared.

【Note】

Exogenous wind cold blocks the exterior resulting in the lung qi failing to disperse, thus resulting in coughing. As the patient has already been ill for ten days there had been some transformation of cold into heat. DU 14 (*dà zhuī*) functions to disperse yang qi thereby relieving exterior symptoms. GB 20 (*fēng chí*) functions to dispel wind and relieve headache. *Tài yáng* (EX-HN5), BL 2 (*cuán zhú*), BL 9 (*yù zhěn*), and GB 20 (*fēng chí*) all treat headache. LI 4 (*hé gǔ*), the *yuán*-source point of the hand *taiyin* lung channel, promotes sweating and resolves the exterior, and LU 7 (*liè quē*), the *luò*-connecting point of the hand *taiyin* lung channel, work together through their interior/exterior relationship to promote diffusion of the lung thus to resolve the exterior. BL 13 (*fèi shù*) promotes diffusion of the lung to stop coughing, and LI 17 (*tiān dǐng*) used together with LU 11 (*shào shāng*) clear heat to treat sore throat.

Bleeding LI 1 (shāng yáng) and LU 11 (shào shāng) using a three-edged needle plus puncturing LI 4 (hé gǔ) with filiform needle and retaining the needle for 30 minutes is a very effective treatment for sore throat.

For carbon monoxide poisoning, in addition to routine treatment, puncturing LU 11 (shào shāng) and DU 26 (rén zhōng) with filiform needle can revive unconscious patients.

Xiao Shao-qing's Medical Record

Zhang, male, 39, first visit was on October 5, 1979

【Chief Complaint】
Headache and fever for 4 days

【Present Medical History】
Four days previously due to not wearing enough clothing, the patient began to experience symptoms of headache, fever, coughing, nasal congestion and pain in the lower back

【Examination】
Throat was red, body temperature of 38.5°C (101.3°F), flabby tongue, with a thin yellow and slightly sticky coating, the pulse was rolling and rapid

【Diagnosis】
Common cold (due to wind heat attacking the lung)

【Treatment Principles】
Dispel wind, clear heat, resolve the exterior

【Treatment】

DU 14 (dà zhuī)	BL 12 (fēng mén)	GB 20 (fēng chí)
BL 13 (fèi shù)	BL 23 (shèn shù)	LI 4 (hé gǔ)

Acupuncture was given once a day with the needles being retained for 20 minutes. After one treatment, the headache and nasal obstruction disappeared, and there was also a reduction in the fever. After two treatments, he was cured.

【Note】
This is influenza. The seasonal epidemic pathogen attacks the lung and blocks the exterior, causing fever and whole body aches. DU 14 (dà

zhuī), the intersection point of all the yang channels, it functions to resolve the exterior by circulating yang qi, additionally it calms the mind and clears heat. BL 23 (*shèn shù*) has a mother/son relationship that facilitates communication between the son (kidney) and the mother (metal), thus producing water to reinforce the body's resistance. BL 12 (*fēng mén*), also knows as *Rè Fǔ* (the left side is called *fēng mén* and the right is known as *Rè Fǔ*), it is the intersection point of *Du mai* and the foot *taiyang* bladder channel, it dispels wind, diffuses the lung, and regulates qi to clear heat. When used together with GB 20 (*fēng chí*), BL 12 (*fēng mén*) has a stronger effect in dispelling wind and resolving the exterior. BL 13 (*fèi shù*), clears the lung, it is used in combination with LI 4 (*hé gǔ*) to resolve the exterior by promoting sweating.

Summary

Common cold, known as injury by wind (*Shāng Fēng* 伤风), includes symptoms of nasal congestion, runny nose and coughing, with chills, fever, and aching throughout the body. It is a common disease seen all year round, but most especially in the winter and spring. It is caused by a deficiency of the normal qi, when there is an invasion of wind cold or wind heat, or a disturbance of the lung's ability to diffuse.

Main points: DU 14 (*dà zhuī*), GB 20 (*fēng chí*), LI 4 (*hé gǔ*).

Tài yáng (EX-HN5), *yìn táng* (EX-HN3), and BL 2 (*cuán zhú*) are added for headache. LU 10 (*yú jì*) or LU 11 (*shào shāng*) are bled to treat sore throat. LU 5 (*chǐ zé*) and LU 9 (*tài yuān*) or BL 13 (*fèi shù*) are added for cough. LI 20 (*yíng xiāng*) is added to clear nasal congestion.

COUGH

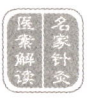

Yang Jie-bin's Medical Record

Fu, female, 27, first visit was on July 29, 1998

【Chief Complaint】

Coughing for one month

【Present Medical History】

The patient's cough began a month ago after she experienced an attack of cold, which resulted in symptoms of dizziness, itchy and sore throat, nasal congestion, runny nose, chills with an aversion to wind, fatigue and full body achiness. The cough was worse at night. Neither taking Western drugs nor an injection of penicillin were helpful. During her visit she coughed repeatedly; the cough had a deep raspy sound, accompanied by white, foamy sputum, which was difficult to expectorate, and chest fullness. Her appetite, urine and stools were all normal.

【Examination】

Pale red tongue, with a thin white coating, pulse was deep and tight

【Diagnosis】

Cough (due to wind cold invasion)

【Treatment Principles】

Promote diffusion of the lung, resolve the exterior, transform phlegm, stop coughing

【Treatment】

①   DU 14 (*dà zhuī*)   GB 20 (*fēng chí*)   LI 4 (*hé gǔ*)

     BL 12 (*fēng mén*)

②   BL 11 (*dà zhù*)   LU 1 (*zhōng fǔ*)   BL 13 (*fèi shù*)

     ST 36 (*zú sān lǐ*)

The above two groups of points were alternately employed once a day, one group each time. Strong reducing stimulation was applied to scatter and disperse the pathogenic wind cold. The needles were retained for 30 minutes after arrival of qi and were restimulated once every 5 minutes using a lifting-thrusting and rotating motion. Cupping was applied after needling at DU 14 (*dà zhuī*), BL 12 (*fēng mén*), BL 11 (*dà zhù*), LU 1 (*zhōng fǔ*), and BL 13 (*fèi shù*) for 15 minutes, which resulted in dark purple marks. After two treatments, the coughing lightened up and sputum was reduced. After four treatments, the cough was almost gone. After six treatments, the cough, expectoration of sputum and fullness in chest basically disappeared. A one month follow-up showed no recurrence.

【Note】

DU 14 (*dà zhuī*) is needed to drain the exterior pathogen from the yang channels. BL 11 (*dà zhù*), GB 20 (*fēng chí*), LI 4 (*hé gǔ*) and BL 12 (*fēng mén*) scatter wind and disperse cold, and diffuse the lung to resolve the exterior. LU 1 (*zhōng fǔ*), the Front-*mù*, and BL 13 (*fèi shù*), the Back-*shù* of the lung, regulate lung qi, transform phlegm and stop coughing. ST 36 (*zú sān lǐ*), the earth point of the foot *yangming* stomach channel, it tonifies the earth to produce the metal, and eliminates dampness and phlegm. These points used together strengthen [the body's] ablity to scatter wind and resolve the exterior, stop coughing and transform phlegm; as the qi moves, phlegm will be accordingly eliminated and the cough will naturally stop.

Records in *Acupuncture - Moxibustion for Difficult Diseases* (*Qí Nán Zá Bìng Zhēn Jiǔ Zhì Liáo*)

Liao, female, 62, first visit was on November 16, 1996

【Chief Complaint】

History of coughing with white phlegm for more than 7 years

【Present Medical History】

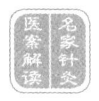

The patient was constitutionally weak and easily caught colds. She often had coughing, chills, fatigue, along with fullness in chest and epigastrium, and loose stools. She had a history of long term use of cough medicines.

【Examination】

Pale tongue, with a white greasy coating, soggy and slippery pulse

【Diagnosis】

Cough (due to phlegm damp retention in the lung)

【Treatment Principles】

Strengthen the spleen to transform dampness and eliminate phlegm to stop coughing

【Treatment】

BL 20 (*pí shù*)	LU 9 (*tài yuān*)	SP 3 (*tài bái*)
LV 13 (*zhāng mén*)	ST 40 (*fēng lóng*)	

Moxibustion was applied to BL 20 (*pí shù*). Other points were needled using a tonifying method. The patient was treated once every other day, she was cured after 30 treatments. Afterwards, blistering moxibustion (***Tiān Jiǔ*** 天灸) was applied once every ten days for six months to consolidate the effect.

【Note】

The spleen fails in transportation and transformation, thus phlegm is produced due to damp retention, which then accumulates in the lung, causing cough with profuse sputum. Spleen deficiency leads to qi deficiency, leading to fatigue and loose stools. Pale tongue, with a white greasy coating, and a soggy and slippery pulse are the signs of phlegm damp. The *yuán*-source points are the places where there is a strong infusion of *zang*-qi, for this reason, LU 9 (*tài yuān*) and SP 3 (*tài bái*) are selected to tonify the lung and spleen. BL 20 (*pí shù*) and LV 13 (*zhāng mén*) are to strengthen and transport the spleen-qi and benefit the lung-qi. ST 40 (*fēng lóng*), *luò*-connecting point of the foot *yangming* stomach channel, strengthens the transport of the stomach and spleen qi in the middle *jiao*, which causes the fluids to disperse, naturally resulting in the transformation of dampness and phlegm.

Tiān Jiǔ (天灸), *is a form of moxibustion, where irritating medicinals are applied to certain acupoints so as to cause blisters. This is often used in the treatment of asthma, chronic bronchitis, allergic rhinitis, chronic cough, weak constitution, susceptibility to common cold, chronic gastroenteritis, insomnia, and pain in low back and legs.*

Zhao, male, 42, his first visit was on April 15, 1958

【Chief Complaint】

Cough for one year and hemoptysis for the previous three days

【Present Medical History】

The patient had been diagnosed with pulmonary tuberculosis a year ago, and was treated with streptomycin and isonicotinyl hydrazide. Presently he was emaciated, spoke with low a voice, coughed up bloody sputum, tidal fever, and night sweating. An injection of a hemostatic medication was not effective for him.

【Examination】

Pale tongue, with a white coating, and thready pulse

【Diagnosis】

Pulmonary tuberculosis with hemoptysis (due to yin deficiency of the lung)

【Treatment Principles】

Tonify yin of the lung to stop bleeding and coughing

【Treatment】

KI 1 (*yǒng quán*)

The patient was treated in the prone position with moxibustion at KI 1 (*yǒng quán*) for 20 minutes, twice a day. After two treatments, the bloody sputum disappeared. With three days of successive treatments, the symptoms basically disappeared. He was advised to continue treatment to fight against the tuberculosis.

【Note】

This is a condition of yin deficiency producing internal heat, moxibustion can be applied in these cases. KI 1 (*yǒng quán*), is the *jǐng*-well point of the Kidney channel, it functions to open orifices, sedate and calm the spirit, is important for blood presentations; through the relation of opposites, it is a point on the lower part of the body that can treat problems in the upper part of the body.

Summary

Cough is known in Chinese as *Ké Sòu* (咳嗽). *Ké* is coughing with sound, but without phlegm; *Sòu* is coughing with phlegm, but without sound. *Ké Sòu* is coughing with both sound and phlegm. It includes coughing from both external attack and internal injury.

Coughing due to external attack is caused by wind, cold, heat and dryness invading the lung. Invasion of wind cold causes cough with thin phlegm, nasal congestion, runny nose, chills, a lack of sweating, thin white tongue coating, and a floating and tight pulse. Invasion of wind heat causes coughing with yellow thick phlegm, feverishness, headache, sweating, aversion to wind, and a floating and rapid pulse. Invasion of dryness and heat causes either a hacking cough or a cough with yellow phlegm that is difficult to expectorate, a dry and sore throat, and a rapid pulse.

Coughing due to internal injury is caused by dysfunctions of the *zang-fu* organs, which often start out as an acute illness, which does not resolve, thus leading to this kind of internal injury. Spleen deficiency produces phlegm damp, fullness in the chest, poor appetite, white greasy coating, and a soft floating pulse; liver fire attacking the lung produces coughing with hypochondriac pain, vomiting, sparse dense sputum, a red face with a dry throat, a yellow coated tongue and wiry rapid pulse; yin deficiency of the lung produces a hacking cough, or coughing with bloody sputum, tidal fever, night sweating, irritability, a hot sensation in the palms and soles, a red tongue, with a sparse coating, and a thready, rapid pulse.

Main points: BL 13 (*fèi shù*), RN 22 (*tiān tū*).

BL 12 (*fēng mén*) and LI 4 (*hé gǔ*) for coughing from external attack. DU 14 (*dà zhuī*) for fever. For bleeding use LU 11 (*shào shāng*). To treat sore throat use LU 5 (*chǐ zé*) and LU 6 (*kǒng zuì*) for coughing of blood. ST 36 (*zú sān lǐ*) and ST 40 (*fēng lóng*) are used for profuse phlegm and poor appetite. GB 34 (*yáng líng quán*) treats hypochondriac pain; for pain or a cold sensation on the back acupuncture can be applied followed by cupping.

ASTHMA

Shao Jing-ming's Medical Records

Zhao, female, 13, first visit was on July 20, 1963

【Chief Complaint】

Asthma for more than 7 years

【Present Medical History】

When she was 6 years old, she had a common cold, which resulted in a lingering cough. In winter her cough would become worse, and it gradually developed into asthma. Presently, regardless of the season no matter whether it was summer or winter, whenever she was exposed to cold she had asthma attacks. During the attack, she had dyspnea, cyanotic lips, wheezing with phlegm in throat and an inability to lie flat.

【Examination】

Emaciated, with cold limbs, pale red tongue, with a white moist and slippery tongue coating, and a deep, thready and forceless pulse

【Diagnosis】

Asthma (due to cold phlegm in the lung)

【Treatment Principles】

Diffuse the lung, transform phlegm, calm wheezing

【Treatment】

DU 14 (*dà zhuī*)	BL 12 (*fēng mén*)	BL 13 (*fèi shù*)

The needles were retained for 15 minutes after arrival of qi; during this time they were manipulated 2-3 times. After removing the needles, moxibustion was applied for 5 to 7 minutes. This treatment eased the

wheezing. This treatment was given once a day. After ten treatments, her breathing was normal. The treatment schedule was changed to every other day after a week of rest. Ten more treatments were given to consolidate the effect. The following winter she did not have any attacks of asthma. When she did get a cold, there was just a bit of chest stuffiness and slight difficulty in breathing. In the following year, she had 20 more acupuncture treatments using the same method. In the third year, she was given another 10 treatments as a consolidation measure. Since then, her constitution was stronger and she no longer had asthma attacks.

【Note】

This patient had an invasion of pathogenic wind when she was small. The pathogen lingered in the lung for a long time, thus bringing about a weakness of *wei* qi, and instability of the exterior; when exposed to wind cold it would result in asthma. DU 14 (*dà zhuī*) diffuses the lung and regulates qi. BL 12 (*fēng mén*) eliminates wind and calms asthma. BL 13 (*fèi shù*) regulates the lung qi and strengthens resistance and stops coughing and wheezing.

Wu, male, 20, first visit was on May 23, 1996

【Chief Complaint】

Asthma for 12 years with a decline in his condition for the previous two years

【Present Medical History】

Twelve years previously, he had a common cold, which induced chest fullness and wheezing. He got better with treatment. But since then, he had had attacks from time to time; in the past two years it had become worse. Treatment with aminophylline and prednisone would give him symptomatic relief, but was not a cure for his bronchial asthma. This last episode lasted for more than one month and previous treatment methods were not effective.

【Examination】

The patient was thin and with a sallow complexion with dyspnea, panting, wheezing with phlegm in the throat, he found it difficult to expectorate the yellow sputum. Auscultation of both lungs revealed rales. His tongue was dark, pale and without moisture. His pulse was rapid and slightly slippery.

【Diagnosis】

Asthma (due to phlegm heat retention)

【Treatment Principles】

Promote the diffusion of the lung, regulate qi, transform phlegm, calm asthma

【Treatment】

| BL 13 (*fèi shù*) | DU 14 (*dà zhuī*) | BL 12 (*fēng mén*) |

With acupuncture treatment he immediately felt relief upon arrival of the qi. Needles were retained for 30 minutes, after removal, his feeling of fullness in chest was greatly improved, but the rales in his lungs were unchanged. After five rounds of the same treatment the asthmatic breathing and wheezing stopped. Two courses (of 20 treatments) made all his symptoms disappear.

【Note】

DU 14 (*dà zhuī*) disperses yang to release the exterior and diffuse the lung to calm asthma. BL 12 (*fēng mén*) dispels pathogens and calms asthma. BL 13 (*fèi shù*) regulates qi of the lung, strengthens the exterior and calms asthma.

Xiao Shao-qing's Medical Record

Zheng, male, 50, first visit was on September 21, 1994

【Chief Complaint】

Coughing and asthma for more than 30 years, in the previous month it had been worse.

【Present Medical History】

He began to have coughing and asthma after he had the measles when he was small. Afterwards, asthma attacks were often induced when he was exposed to cold or ate seafood. One month ago, his condition worsened after getting chilled. Use of an inhaler gave some symptomatic relief but, he had symptoms of coughing and wheezing, with fullness and pain in the chest which was worse at night, profuse white sticky phlegm that was difficult to expectorate, and was thirsty with a desire to drink. His appetite, urine and stools were normal.

【Examination】

Rough breathing, rales, pale tongue, with a white sticky coating, and a thin, wiry and slippery pulse

【Diagnosis】

Asthma (due to invasion of wind cold, phlegm damp in the lung)

【Treatment Principles】

Scatter wind cold from the lung, transform phlegm, stop coughing and calm asthma

【Treatment】

RN 17 (*dàn zhōng*)	RN 22 (*tiān tū*)	*dìng chuǎn* (EX-B1)
ST 40 (*fēng lóng*)	PC 6 (*nèi guān*)	LI 4 (*hé gǔ*)
LU 7 (*liè quē*)		

RN 22 (*tiān tū*) was needled with a three inch filiform needle, which was inserted perpendicularly and obliquely along the posterior border of the manubrium of the sternum to a depth of about 2.5 inches; the point was stimulated with a twisting motion and then the needle was immediately withdrawn. RN 17 (*dàn zhōng*) was also needled with a three inch filiform needle, which was obliquely inserted to the depth about 2.5 inches and rotated while lifting and thrusting to produce a strong sensation. Other points were needled with an even method and then retained for 20 minutes;

needles were stimluated once every 10 minutes. Treatment was given on a daily basis.

On the second visit, the patient's coughing, wheezing, and chest pain showed signs of improvement. He was able to lie flat at night, and the sputum, while still profuse was easy to expectorate. Therefore, the previous treatment was applied again.

On the sixth visit, his coughing and wheezing had ceased, the sputum had become thin and sparse, and the rales were reduced. It was thought that the lingering pathogenic factors had been expelled, but the normal qi was still weak. BL 13 (*fèi shù*) and BL 23 (*shèn shù*) were used instead of LI 4 (*hé gǔ*) and LU 7 (*liè quē*). Acupuncture with a tonifying method, cupping and moxibustion were applied at RN 4 (*guān yuán*) and RN 6 (*qì hǎi*). One more course of treatment cured him completely.

【Note】

The patient had suffered from asthma for 30 years, due to the length of this illness it was thought his lung, spleen and kidney surely must be weak thus invasion of wind cold disturbed the lung's ability to diffuse. Due to qi deficiency of lung, spleen and kidney the water metabolism became disordered, thereby producing phlegm dampness. In the acute stage, the branch symptom (*Biāo* 标) of wheezing should be immediately brought under control. For this purpose, RN 17 (*dàn zhōng*), RN 22 (*tiān tū*) and *dìng chuǎn* (EX-B1) were selected to descend qi to stop coughing and wheezing. PC 6 (*nèi guān*) was needled to regulate qi and relieve fullness and pain in the chest. ST 40 (*fēng lóng*) was used to transform phlegm. LU 7 (*liè quē*) and LI 4 (*hé gǔ*), is a combination of *yuán* and *luò* points, used together they scatter cold and eliminate wind. After the acute symptoms were relieved, the root cause (*Běn* 本) was treated by using BL 13 (*fèi shù*) and BL 23 (*shèn shù*) to tonify the generative cycle between the lung and kidney, and using RN 4 (*guān yuán*) and RN 6 (*qì hǎi*) to support and firm up the original qi. Moxibustion and cupping were important methods in the treatment for this case.

Summary

Asthma is an allergic disease of the respiratory tract. Characterized by repeated attacks of paroxysmal dyspnea with wheezing, it is difficult to treat. Professor Shao Jing-ming is experienced in treating such a disease. According to him, asthma is due to both the [root cause (*Běn*本)] of an underlying weakness in resistance due to a deficiency of the *zang-fu* organs, along with [branch (*Biāo*标)] excess due to invasion of external pathogens. The former refers to hypofunction of the lung, spleen and kidney and the latter to phlegm, dampness, blood stasis and external invasion. Promoting the lung's function of diffusion, regulating qi, and transforming phlegm are the principles to follow for its treatment.

Main points: DU 14 (*dà zhuī*), BL 12 (*fēng mén*), BL 13 (*fèi shù*).

As proven by the clinical practice, BL 13 (*fèi shù*) is on the foot *taiyang* bladder channel, it is a special point on the back that is infused with lung qi, this point is good at regulating the qi and strengthening resistance to stop coughing and wheezing. DU 14 (*dà zhuī*) also called the "meeting point of yang" is good to disperse yang qi to disperse wind cold and descend qi to calm asthma. BL 12 (*fēng mén*) is the meeting point of the foot *tài yáng* and Du channels which is used to disperse wind cold, drain heat pathogens, and regulate qi of the lung to stop coughing and wheezing; moxibustion on this point can stimulate the channel qi, consolidate exterior and prevent the common cold.

During an asthma attack, these three points used together can reduce pressure in the lower respiratory tract. When used in the acute stage, they improve the functioning of lungs. They are especially effective for bronchial asthma.

Points for symptomatic treatment: LI 4 (*hé gǔ*) is added for treating external pathogens. LU 5 (*chǐ zé*) and LU 9 (*tài yuān*) treat coughing. RN 12 (*zhōng wǎn*) and ST 36 (*zú sān lǐ*) are used for profuse phlegm. RN 22 (*tiān tū*) and RN 17 (*dàn zhōng*) for phlegm blockage of the windpipe. BL 23 (*shèn shù*), RN 4 (*guān yuán*) and KI 3 (*tài xī*) for asthma of a deficiency type. BL 14 (*jué yīn shù*), BL 15 (*xīn shù*) and PC 6 (*nèi guān*) treat palpitations. LU 10 (*yú jì*) treats dry throat. LU 10 (*yú jì*), LU 6 (*kǒng zuì*) and LU 5 (*chǐ zé*) for hemoptysis. RN 12 (*zhōng wǎn*), ST 36 (*zú sān lǐ*), ST 25 (*tiān shū*) and RN 6 (*qì hǎi*) are used to treat epigastric fullness. SP 9 (*yīn líng quán*), ST 28 (*shuǐ dào*) and ST 36 (*zú sān lǐ*) are effective for edema of lower limbs.

Treatment should be given once a day during the acute stage and every other day when in the non-acute stage. Ten acupuncture sessions are considered one course of treatment. For adults, 1 inch needles are inserted to 0.5~0.8 inches in depth. For children, 0.5 inch needles are inserted to a depth of 0.2~0.3 inches. Needles are retained for half an hour and stimulated one or twice during that time.

Application of tonifying or draining techniques are in accord with the patient's individual condition. For children less than one year old, do not retain the needles. Moxibustion and cupping are used accordingly.

HYPOCHONDRIAC PAIN

Cheng Xin-nong's Medical Records

Xu, male, 47, first visit was on July 25, 1987

【Chief Complaint】

Chest discomfort for more than 2 years

【Present Medical History】

When fatigued the patient would have fullness and pain in the chest. Recently, there was an aggravation of the pain and it radiated to the back and arm. Neither bed rest nor treatment with glonoin brought him relief. The patient reported feeling tired, short of breath, with a cold feeling in the low back, and abdominal distention after eating. His sleep was not good; urine was yellow.

【Examination】

Dark lips with petechiae, blood pressure was normal at 120/80mm Hg, dark tongue, slightly thick coating, pulse was wiry, thin and rough with missed beats

【Diagnosis】

Obstruction of qi in the chest (*Xiōng Bì* 胸痹) (qi deficiency and blood stasis)

【Treatment Principles】

Tonify the qi, dredge channels and collaterals

【Treatment】

DU 14 (*dà zhuī*)	RN 17 (*dàn zhōng*)	RN 12 (*zhōng wǎn*)
RN 6 (*qì hǎi*)	PC 6 (*nèi guān*)	LU 9 (*tài yuān*)
ST 36 (*zú sān lǐ*)	SP 6 (*sān yīn jiāo*)	LI 15 (*jiān yú*) (*left*)

All points were needled with even method.

【Note】

This patient is constitutionally weak in yang qi, so there is a feeling cold in low back and abdomen distention after eating. Yang qi deficiency in chest leads to blood stasis, so there is chest pain and discomfort. DU 14 (*dà zhuī*), is the intersection point of all the yang channels; it effectively circulates yang qi. RN 17 (*dàn zhōng*), is the meeting point of qi and Front-*mù* of the pericardium, it regulates the qi of the heart and stops pain. RN 12 (*zhōng wǎn*), the meeting point of the *fu* organs and the Front-*mù* of the stomach, it strengthens the spleen and stomach, invigorates qi and blood, tonifies the qi of the middle *jiao*, and calms the mind. RN 6 (*qì hǎi*) enhances the kidney and the primal qi. ST 36 (*zú sān lǐ*) tonifies and nourishes the spleen and stomach and supports post-natal qi. PC 6 (*nèi guān*) strengthens the heart, stabilizes the will and invigorates the channels to stop pain. LU 9 (*tài yuān*), the meeting point of the vessels, is used together with PC 6 (*nèi guān*) and SP 6 (*sān yīn jiāo*) to tonify qi, open the yang to get rid of blood stasis and open the channels. LI 15 (*jiān yú*) opens the channels and collaterals, and circulates qi and blood to stop pain.

Zheng, male, 58, first visit was on November 4, 1985

【Chief Complaint】

Left hypochondriac pain for 3 days

【Present Medical History】

The patient is bad-tempered and easily angered, a few days ago he had a quarrel with somebody. Afterwards, he lost his appetite, and had abdominal distention and acid regurgitation. Three days ago he suddenly had a pain in the left hypochondrium, which was made worse with coughing.

【Examination】

No obvious swelling in the left hypochondrium but there was tenderness, the tongue was pale with a thick greasy yellow coating, along with a wiry pulse.

【Diagnosis】

Hypochondriac pain (due to liver qi stagnation)

【Treatment Principles】

Calm the the liver, regulate qi, open the channels, stop pain

【Treatment】

GB 34 (*yáng líng quán*)	LV 3 (*tài chōng*)	ST 36 (*zú sān lǐ*)
SJ 6 (*zhī gōu*)	LV 14 (*qī mén*) (left)	

These points were needled with a draining method. After the treatment, the patient immediately felt much better and his appetite gradually returned and the abdominal distension and tenderness were reduced. After four rounds of the above treatment, he was cured.

【Note】

This patient's habitual bad temper was damaging to his liver and resulted in qi stagnation in channels running to the hypochondria, thus there was distention and pain. The *Miraculous Pivot* (*Líng Shū*, 灵枢) says: "If there is a pathogen in the liver, there will be pain in the hypochondria". LV 14 (*qī mén*), the Front-*mù* of liver, LV 3 (*tài chōng*), the *yuán*-source point of liver, together with GB 34 (*yáng líng quán*), *hé*-sea of the gall bladder, are used to regulate the liver-qi, and together with SJ 6 (*zhī gōu*), work to dredge the channels and smooth the qi mechanism, thus opening the channels and smoothing the flow of qi and blood, with free flow there is no pain (通则不痛 *tōng zé bù tòng*). ST 36 (*zú sān lǐ*) is to strengthen the spleen and open the stomach, use of this point helped to improve his appetite and reduce the abdominal distension.

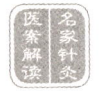

Yang Jie-bin's Medical Record

Chen, female, 63

【Chief Complaint】

Right hypochondriac pain for 20 days

【Present Medical History】

Twenty days before, at night, she suddenly had a serious pain in the right hypochondriac region, which radiated to the back and was made worse with coughing and even breathing. She hurried to the emergency room and the x-ray examination showed no abnormalities with her heart and lungs. Administered a pain killer, sleeping pill, gentamicin (an antibiotic), and various herbal medicines, none of which brought her any relief. Now, in addition to the previous symptoms, she has dizziness, tinnitus, and dry throat.

【Previous Diagnosis】

Hypertension

【Examination】

Red face, strong constitution, troubled expression with a moaning voice, restlessness, tenderness in the area from the 3rd to 7th rib, slightly red tongue, sparse coating, wiry and tight pulse

【Diagnosis】

Hypochondriac pain

【Treatment Principles】

Open the channels and invigorate collaterals, regulate qi circulation, stop pain

【Treatment】

Right side:	SJ 6 (*zhī gōu*)	GB 34 (*yáng líng quán*)
	ST 18 (*rǔ gēn*)	PC 1 (*tiān chí*)

SJ 6 (*zhī gōu*) was needled through to PC 5 (*jiān shǐ*) with #28 2 inch filiform needle using strong stimulation to drain, GB 34 (*yáng líng quán*) and SP 9 (*yīn líng quán*) were needled in a similar fashion. The needles were retained for half an hour, during which time they were manipulated with lifting-thrusting and rotating once every 3 minutes. Cupping was applied to ST 18 (*rǔ gēn*) and PC 1 (*tiān chí*) for 15 minutes.

The pain stopped within twenty minutes and the patient was cured after this half hour treatment. The follow-up showed no recurrence of hypochondriac pain.

【Note】

SJ 6 (*zhī gōu*) is the fire point on the hand *shaoyang sanjiao* channel. Needling this point adjusts the qi of the channel and reduces the ministerial fire. GB 34 (*yáng líng quán*), the *hé*-sea point on the foot *shaoyang* gallbladder channel, treats *fu* organs to adjusts the qi of the fu organs, invigorates the collaterals to stop pain. Cupping on ST 18 (*rǔ gēn*) and PC 1 (*tiān chí*) removes local blood stasis to stop pain.

Summary

Chest and hypochondriac pain is due to qi stagnation and blood stasis. The heart yang is inactive and the lung qi is constrained, or overeating cold food causes cold accumulating in the middle *jiao* with counterflow rising up to the chest, this produces obstruction of the channels in the chest region, thereby resulting in chest and hypochondriac pain.

Main points: RN 17 (*dàn zhōng*), PC 7 (*dà líng*), LU 9 (*tài yuān*), PC 6 (*nèi guān*).

Add DU 14 (*dà zhuī*) and BL 15 (*xīn shù*) to activate the heart yang. Add BL 13 (*fèi shù*), LU 1 (*zhōng fǔ*) and LU 7 (*liè quē*) to diffuse the lung qi. Add RN 22 (*tiān tū*) and ST 40 (*fēng lóng*) to transform phlegm. Apply moxibustion at BL 13 (*fèi shù*), BL 15 (*xīn shù*) and RN 17 (*dàn zhōng*) after needling to relieve pain that radiates to the back and to dispel cold due to excessive yin. Add LV 2 (*xíng jiān*), SP 10 (*xuè hǎi*), LI 4 (*hé gǔ*), SP 6 (*sān yīn jiāo*) to activate qi and improve blood circulation for those prolonged cases with qi stagnation and blood stasis.

Hypochondriac pain is related to liver and gallbladder diseases and further connected with the course of the *shaoyang* channels. In the *Miraculous Pivot - Five Pathogenic Factors (Líng Shū: Wǔ Xié, 灵枢 • 五邪)* it says: "When the pathogen is in the liver, there will be pain in the hypochondria" *Miraculous Pivot - Channels*

(*Líng Shū: Jīng Mài*, 灵枢 • 经脉) says: "The patients with gallbladder diseases will have a bitter taste in the mouth, sigh frequently, suffer from pain in the heart and hypochondriac regions, and have difficulty in turning the body."

Intercostal neuralgia and pleurisy and hypochondriac pain caused by traumatic injury can be treated with the principle mentioned here.

Main points: GB 34 (*yáng líng quán*), SJ 6 (*zhī gōu*), LV 14 (*qī mén*).

Hypochondriac pain due to liver qi stagnation has symptoms of distending pain, chest fullness, bitter taste in the mouth and a wiry pulse; to treat add points such as BL 18 (*gān shù*), BL 19 (*dǎn shù*) and GB 40 (*qiū xū*).

For hypochondriac pain due to blood stasis caused by trauma with symptoms such as stabbing pain, especially at night, along with stasis spots on the tongue and a wiry rough pulse; add BL 17 (*gé shù*) and LV 3 (*tài chōng*).

For hypochondriac pain which is due to phlegm retention caused by prolonged coughing and damp retained in the chest and hypochondria with symptoms such as dyspnea, white moist tongue coating and thin soggy pulse, RN 12 (*zhōng wǎn*), ST 36 (*zú sān lǐ*) and BL 20 (*pí shù*) should be added.

EPIGASTRIC PAIN

Cheng Xin-nong's Medical Records

Yan, male, 29, first visit was on December 2, 1985

【Chief Complaint】

Pain in the epigastric region for 7 years

【Present Medical History】

The patient began to have pain fixed in the epigastric region seven years ago. He was diagnosed with a duodenal ulcer, however the medicinal treatment he had received was not effective. He would experience a fixed indistinct dull pain that usually started one to two hours after eating and would be relieved by pressure. He preferred warm drinks. His appetite was normal, no nausea or vomiting. His urine and stools were normal.

【Examination】

Sallow complexion, tip of tongue red, with a slightly yellow coating, the pulse was weak wiry

【Diagnosis】

Epigastric pain (due to cold stagnation in the stomach)

【Treatment Principles】

Warm the middle *jiao*, dispel cold, circulate qi, stop pain

【Treatment】

RN 12 (*zhōng wǎn*)	RN 6 (*qì hǎi*)	PC 6 (*nèi guān*)
SP 4 (*gōng sūn*)	ST 36 (*zú sān lǐ*)	SP 6 (*sān yīn jiāo*)

Tonifying and even methods were applied. Moxibustion was applied to RN 12 (*zhōng wǎn*). After one treatment, he reported feeling better. He was treated once daily for 10 consecutive days, after which the pain disappeared.

【Note】

In this case, the spleen and stomach both were diseased, due to a deficiency of yang in the middle *jiao*, the stomach qi was not harmonized, thus pain in the epigastric region. RN 12 (*zhōng wǎn*), the Front-*mù* of the stomach, was used to harmonize the stomach by warming the yang to dispel cold. ST 36 (*zú sān lǐ*), Lower *hé*-sea of the foot *yangming* stomach channel, was used with SP 6 (*sān yīn jiāo*) the intersection point of the lower leg yin channels, to strengthen the stomach and construct the spleen. SP 4 (*gōng sūn*) is the *luò*-connecting point of the foot *taiyin* spleen channel, needling with PC 6 (*nèi guān*) of the pericardium channel connects them through the *yinwei mai*; they function to relax the chest, regulate the qi and harmonize the stomach.

Run, female, 60, first visit was on April 6, 1992

【Chief Complaint】

Pain in the epigastrium for 10 years

【Present Medical History】

Due to distending pain in the epigastrium this patient had an ultrasound examination and was subsequently given the diagnosis of cholecystitis. Ultrasound findings show she had a 0.6cm ×1.5cm stone in the gall bladder and a 1.4cm cyst on the right lobe of the liver. She experienced pain in the hypochondria, which would be accompanied by hiccups; symptoms could be relieved by warmth. She sometimes had palpitations. Her stools were loose.

【Examination】

Lusterless complexion, purple tongue with a thin yellow coating, right pulse was deep and thin, left pulse deep wiry.

【Diagnosis】

Epigastric pain (due to Liver qi attacking Stomach)

【Treatment Principles】

Dredge the Liver, regulate qi, harmonize the stomach, stop pain

【Treatment】

RN 17 (dàn zhōng)	RN 12 (zhōng wǎn)	RN 6 (qì hǎi)
GB 24 (rì yuè)	PC 6 (nèi guān)	BL 21 (wèi shù)
BL 19 (dǎn shù)	GB 34 (yáng líng quán)	ST 36 (zú sān lǐ)
LV 3 (tài chōng)	GB 40 (qiū xū)	

Draining and even methods were applied. The distending pain in the epigastrium was gradually relieved and after 40 treatments she was cured.

【Note】

Feelings of depression stagnates liver qi, causing the liver qi to counterflow and attack the Earth organs, because the liver and stomach are out of harmony the turbid fails to properly descend, thus causing distending pain, hiccups and loose, but incomplete stools. Long-term constraint transforms into fire, involving the qi and blood, thus the purple tongue with yellow coating. RN 12 (*zhōng wǎn*) and BL 21 (*wèi shù*), GB 24 (*rì yuè*) and BL 19 (*dǎn shù*) is a combination of Front-*mù* and Back-*shù* points that harmonize the stomach, dredge the liver, and regulate qi to stop pain. BL 19 (*dǎn shù*), GB 34 (*yáng líng quán*), LV 3 (*tài chōng*), and GB 40 (*qiū xū*) function to descend the upward rushing of liver qi thus helping to harmonize the stomach. PC 6 (*nèi guān*) and RN 17 (*dàn zhōng*) relax the chest and circulate qi. ST 36 (*zú sān lǐ*), RN 12 (*zhōng wǎn*) and PC 6 (*nèi guān*) harmonize the stomach to stop pain. RN 6 (*qì hǎi*) consolidates *yuán*-source qi and harmonizes qi and blood.

Tian Cong-huo's Medical Record

X X, female, 34, first visit was on November 23, 2005

【Chief Complaint】

Repeated distending pain in the upper abdomen for two years, worse for one month

【Present Medical History】

Two years ago, this patient for no apparent reason had a distending pain in the upper abdomen, which was diagnosed as a duodenal ulcer. Medicinal treatment with a combination of Chinese and Western medicine was not effective. In the past month the pain became worse. After eating she would have bloating, acid regurgitation, belching, and a dislike of cold. She had one or two loose bowel movements every day; urine was yellow.

【Examination】

Gastroscopy showed there to be chronic superficial gastritis and weak peristalsis. The pathological findings included moderate chronic atrophic gastritis at the antral region, interstitial congestion, and glandular hyperplasia. She had a pale red tongue with a yellow greasy coating, and a

thin, wiry pulse.

【Diagnosis】

Epigastric pain (due to damp heat retention in the middle *jiao*, Liver qi stagnation)

【Treatment Principles】

Adjust the qi mechanism, open and benefit the *sanjiao*.

【Treatment】

DU 14 (*dà zhuī*)	DU 6 (*jǐ zhōng*)	RN 12 (*zhōng wǎn*)
ST 21 (*liáng mén*)	ST 36 (*zú sān lǐ*)	PC 6 (*nèi guān*)
LV 14 (*qī mén*)	KI 16 (*huāng shù*)	BL 20 (*pí shù*)
BL 21 (*wèi shù*)		

To unobstruct the *du* vessel, an ***elongated needle*** (*máng zhēn* 芒针) 380 mm in length was used to needle from DU 14 (*dà zhuī*) through to DU 6 (*jǐ zhōng*). RN 12 (*zhōng wǎn*), ST 21 (*liáng mén*), ST 36 (*zú sān lǐ*), PC 6 (*nèi guān*), LV 14 (*qī mén*), and KI 16 (*huāng shù*) were also needled. Cupping was applied at BL 20 (*pí shù*) and BL 21 (*wèi shù*).

The patient was treated three times a week, the long *máng zhēn* was used once a week; when the symptoms improved it was changed to a short *máng zhēn* and used less frequently. Other points were selected and needled accordingly.

With nearly two months' treatment, the symptoms disappeared and the gastroscope showed that her chronic superficial gastritis had been cured.

【Note】

The *du* vessel connects with all the yang channels at DU 14 (*dà zhuī*). The *dai* - girdling vessel originates from the second lumbar vertebra. The *yangwei mai* meets the *du* vessel at DU 16 (*fēng fǔ*) and DU 15 (*yǎ mén*). The *yangqiao mai* connects with DU 16 (*fēng fǔ*) through the foot *taiyang* bladder channel. The *du* vessel, connects with the kidney which stores the original yang, and with all yang channels, the yang qi circulates externally and protects the body from invasion by external pathogenic factors; internally it warms the *zang-fu* organs, and plays a role in the formation of essence and blood. According to Professor Tian Cong-huo, the *du* vessel is responsible for yang diseases anywhere in the body, or for illness in any one of yang channels. Regulating the *du* vessel with an elongated needle that connects multiple points produces fast results, but because it is a strong treatment, it can be used only once a week or less. For this patient, the use of the elongated needle produced excellent effect in promoting the circulation of qi by adjusting the qi mechanism and opening the *sanjiao*; thus eliminating the symptoms of damp heat caused by stagnant liver qi.

Elongated Needle (*máng zhēn* 芒针) **Regulating** *Du Vessel*:

The position of the patient is extremely important when using this method; they should either be in lying prone, in a lateral recumbent position, or sitting erect with their back towards the doctor. Professor Tian's Elongated needle (máng zhēn) technique consists of a quick insertion of the needle by grasping it near the tip, and using a flick of the wrist of the needling hand to pierce the skin. The needling hand then acts to insert the needle down along the posterior border of the spine, while the supporting hand controls the direction of the needle. Once the tip of the needle reaches its destination it can be manipulated to tonify or drain. In the interest of safety it is suggested to supplement or drain by means of respiration, rotating or rapid and slow insertion and withdrawal, not lifting-thrusting. To supplement ask the patient to inhale while manipulating the needle with the thumb by turning it forward, and closing the hole when withdrawing. To reduce, do the opposite. The rotation should be gentle and agile with an amplitude of 180°~360°. The 125~175 mm elongated needle may be retained for 20 minutes. The longer ones, of 380 mm, 500 mm, or 1200 mm are not retained. The needle should be kept straight when withdrawing in order to prevent difficulties in removal; violent withdrawal should be avoided.

Shao Jing-ming's Medical Record

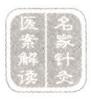

Liu, female, 29, first visit was on June 25, 1999

【Chief Complaint】
Stomach pain and abdominal distention for 5 months

【Present Medical History】

One year previously she began to have discomfort in the upper abdomen; sometimes a bearing-down distention. In the past five months due to being busy she did not have time to eat on a regular basis this resulted in stomach pain. Metoclopramide helped to mitigate the pain, but did not control it. She experienced symptoms of abdominal distension, poor appetite, fatigue, and poor sleep. The provincial hospital used a barium examination and diagnosed her with prolapse of the stomach (Ⅱ). The treatment she had previously received was not effective.

【Examination】

The patient had a thin build, pale complexion which lacked luster, her spirit was fine, her abdomen pouched out and was tender with palpation, the tongue was pale with a thin coating, and a deep, slow pulse.

【Diagnosis】

Prolapse of the stomach (due to yang deficiency)

【Treatment Principles】

Strengthen the spleen, harmonize the stomach, lift and raise yang qi

【Treatment】

RN 12 (zhōng wǎn)	ST 36 (zú sān lǐ)	wèi shàng (EX-CA2)
PC 6 (nèi guān)	HT 7 (shén mén)	SP 6 (sān yīn jiāo)

The patient was treated once a day, after six treatments, her appetite and sleep improved, as did her energy level. Afterwards the main points RN 12 (zhōng wǎn), ST 36 (zú sān lǐ), and wèi shàng (EX-CA2) were needled every other day. After two courses of treatment, her symptoms disappeared and an x-ray examination showed that the stomach returned to normal position. One year follow-up did not manifest any recurrence.

【Note】

Prolapse of the stomach is commonly seen in clinic. Professor Shao holds that it is mostly caused by irregular food intake, fatigue due to overwork, prolonged illness, or childbirth which weakens the constitution and exhausts the spleen yang, resulting in the qi of the middle *jiao* being too weak to hold the organs in place. The main points are RN 12 (*zhōng wǎn*), ST 36 (*zú sān lǐ*), *wèi shàng* (EX-CA2). The points for symptomatic relief include: PC 6 (*nèi guān*) for poor appetite, nausea and acid regurgitation; BL 20 (*pí shù*) and BL 21 (*wèi shù*) for abdominal distension; DU 20 (*bǎi huì*) for bearing-down sensation in abdomen and diarrhea; HT 7 (*shén mén*) and SP 6 (*sān yīn jiāo*) for insomnia. For those with yang deficiency, apply moxibustion.

> **Wèi shàng** (EX-CA2), *located 2 inches above the umbilicus and 4 inches lateral to the anterior midline, it functions to rapidly reinforce qi, strengthen the spleen, and lift the stomach, it is a good point for treating prolapse of the stomach. A 3~4 inches filiform needle is used, inserted obliquely towards RN 8 (shén què) to a depth 2.5~3.5 inches into the muscle. A medium strong stimulation is applied to produce a lifting and contracting sensation in the epigastric region. The direction and depth are important. Treatment should be given on an empty stomach. If the patient feels pain and discomfort from the treatment, they should rest for a while afterwards.*

Summary

Stomach pain is common in cases of peptic ulcer, acute and chronic gastritis, and nervous stomach. It is often caused by irregular food intake, invasion of cold or depression. Upper abdominal pain is often accompanied by nausea, vomiting, abdominal distension, and belching. It may be worse under pressure or could be better by applying warmth and pressure. The deep and slippery pulse points to an excess condition, while a deep, thin and wiry pulse suggests a deficiency syndrome. The treating strategy is to harmonize the stomach to stop pain.

Main points: RN 12 (*zhōng wǎn*), ST 36 (*zú sān lǐ*), PC 6 (*nèi guān*).

For distending pain due to food retention use: ST 21 (*liáng mén*), ST 44 (*nèi tíng*), SP 4 (*gōng sūn*).

Cold stagnation in the stomach resulting in the vomiting of clear fluids, with pain that is relieved by warmth, and a slow pulse apply moxibustion on: BL 20 (*pí shù*), BL 21 (*wèi shù*), RN 6 (*qì hǎi*).

Liver attacking the stomach leading to hypochondriac pain needle: GB 34 (*yáng líng quán*), LV 3 (*tài chōng*).

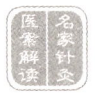

HICCUP

Yang Jie-bin's Medical Record

Yang, male, 30

【Chief Complaint】
Loud hiccups for more than 10 days

【Present Medical History】
Eleven days ago the patient began to have loud non-stop hiccupping after lunch, which was accompanied by abdominal distention, chest stuffiness, acid regurgitation, and headache, all of which made the patient tired. The patient was treated with both oral administration and injections of muscle relaxants, as well as sedatives and fiber, all were ineffective.

【Examination】
The patient was in robust health, but he had a pained expression, the continuous hiccupping made talking and breathing difficult, his tongue had a thin white coating, and his pulse was wiry and slippery.

【Diagnosis】
Hiccups

【Treatment Principles】
Relax the chest, smooth qi circulation, harmonize the middle *jiao*

【Treatment】

RN 17 (*dàn zhōng*)	BL 17 (*gé shù*)	GB 20 (*fēng chí*)
PC 6 (*nèi guān*)	C3~4 *jiá jǐ* (EX-B2)	ST 36 (*zú sān lǐ*)

RN 17 (*dàn zhōng*) was needled through to RN 16 (*zhōng tíng*), BL 17 (*gé shù*) was needled obliquely 1.5 inches toward the spine, PC 6 (*nèi guān*) was needled through to SJ 5 (*wài guān*), *jiá jǐ* (EX-B2) was obliquely needled 1.5 inches towards the spine, RN 12 (*zhōng wǎn*) and ST 36 (*zú sān lǐ*) were needled in a standard fashion.

Both needling and cupping were used. Ten minutes later, the hiccuping had decreased and half an hour later it stopped. The patient slept 10 hours that day. One more treatment was given on the following day to consolidate the good result of the previous treatment. There were no recurrences after one week.

【Note】

Hiccups are due to an abnormal rising of qi. RN 17 (*dàn zhōng*) and BL 17 (*gé shù*) relax the chest to smooth the qi mechinsim. RN 12 (*zhōng wǎn*), the Influential point of *fu* organs and Front-*mù* of the stomach, harmonizes the stomach and sends qi downward. PC 6 (*nèi guān*) needled through to SJ 5 (*wài guān*), should send a sensation into the chest that then directly regulates the qi activities of the *sanjiao*. ST 36 (*zú sān lǐ*), *hé*-sea point, regulates the qi of stomach. *Jiá jǐ* (EX-B2) comforts the chest to stop hiccups.

Summary

Hiccups are often caused by a disturbance of the stomach due to improper eating, which results in a failure of the qi to descend. Professor Yang Jie-bin utilizes the principle of harmonizing the stomach to descend the qi.

Main points: RN 17 (*dàn zhōng*), BL 17 (*gé shù*), RN 12 (*zhōng wǎn*), PC 6 (*nèi guān*).

Assisted points: C3~4 *jiá jǐ* (EX-B2), ST 36 (*zú sān lǐ*).

A combination of local and distal points are used in this treatment. A #28 filiform needle is used to give strong dispersing. Needles are retained for half an hour, with a lifting-thrusting and rotating stimulation given once every three minutes. Arrival of qi is a must! After needling, cupping should be applied. Generally, this treatment brings rapid relief. For mild cases, needling of just PC 6 (*nèi guān*) or *jiá jǐ* (EX-B2) may immediately stop the hiccuping. When the usual points are not effective, pressing or needling SJ 17 (*yì fēng*) can be remarkably helpful.

ABDOMINAL PAIN

Feng Run-shen's Medical Record

Fan, male, 37

【Chief Complaint】

Abdominal pain with an upward rushing sensation from below the umbilicus

【Present Medical History】

The patient began to experience abdominal distention after eating something cold. The pain started after he went to bed, there was feeling of distention with an upward rushing sensation from below the umbilicus, once every three to fives minutes. It became worse at midnight and caused him to sweat profusely. Afterwards he vomited and had thirst with a preference for warm drinks. He had scanty urination and had been constipated for the previous two days.

【Examination】

The patient had a greenish yellow complexion, purple lips, cold extremities, abdominal muscle tension and the pain was made worse with pressure, the tongue had a thin dry coating, and the pulse was thin, wiry and rapid, and weak at the bottom.

【Diagnosis】

Running piglet syndrome (奔豚 bēn tún) abdominal pain (due to cold qi being forced upward)

【Treatment Principles】

Warm and tonify the spleen and kidney, dispel cold, descend counterflow

【Treatment】

RN 4 (*guān yuán*)	ST 36 (*zú sān lǐ*)	SP 6 (*sān yīn jiāo*)
KI 6 (*zhào hǎi*)	LV 3 (*tài chōng*)	

These points were needled with a tonifying method and the pain was immediately relieved. Needle moxa was used to deeply warm the points. About 10 minutes later, the pain was completely relieved.

【Note】

This is a case of constitutional kidney yang deficiency. The consumption of cold food forces cold qi from lower *jiao* to run upward, thus causing pain and the sensation of something running upward to the chest. RN 4 (*guān yuán*) is used to warm the lower *jiao*, ST 36 (*zú sān lǐ*) is needled to strengthen the spleen and stomach, SP 6 (*sān yīn jiāo*) warms and moves the spleen yang and restores the kidney yang, LV 3 (*tài chōng*) and KI 6 (*zhào hǎi*) to subdue the ascension of liver qi. The pain stops due to the spleen yang being warmed, and kidney qi strengthened; when the cold is dispelled and counterflow qi descended, the pain is reduced naturally.

Cheng Xin-nong's Medical Record

Jin, male, 25, first visit was on January 21, 1984

【Chief Complaint】

Colicky pain in the umbilical region for one year

【Present Medical History】

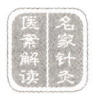

Beginning one year ago, about once a month the patient would experience a paroxysmal colicky pain in the periumbilical region which would last for about 10 hours, and was accompanied by nausea and vomiting. Additionally he suffered from ascariasis. His appetite and sleep were both poor, daily bowel movements, but the stool was dry, urination was normal.

【Examination】

White tongue coat, tip of the tongue was red, the pulse was deep, thin and wiry

【Diagnosis】

Abdominal pain

【Treatment Principles】

Warm the middle *jiao*, tonify the spleen and stomach, regulate qi to stop pain

【Treatment】

PC 6 (*nèi guān*)	SP 4 (*gōng sūn*)	ST 36 (*zú sān lǐ*)
SP 6 (*sān yīn jiāo*)	RN 10 (*xià wǎn*)	RN 6 (*qì hǎi*)
ST 25 (*tiān shū*)		

Moxibustion was applied to ST 25 (*tiān shū*) and an even method acupuncture was applied to the other points.

【Note】

This abdominal pain related to ascariasis, which is a chronic disorder of the qi mechanism. The principle here is to warm the middle *jiao*, tonify the spleen and stomach, and regulate qi to stop the pain.

Summary

Abdominal pain refers to the pain in the area below the xiphoid process and above the pubis. The divergent channels of the foot *taiyin* and foot *yangming* enter into the abdomen, the liver channel also enters into lower abdomen, as does the *ren* vessel which runs through the interior of the abdomen. Abdominal pain is often related to these four channels.

Main points: RN 12 (*zhōng wǎn*), ST 25 (*tiān shū*), ST 36 (*zú sān lǐ*), SP 6 (*sān yīn jiāo*), LV 3 (*tài chōng*).

RN 8 (*shén què*) and SP 4 (*gōng sūn*) are used together to treat retention of cold in the interior. SP 9 (*yīn líng quán*) is coupled with ST 44 (*nèi tíng*) to treat stagnation due to damp heat. RN 4 (*guān yuán*), BL 20 (*pí shù*), BL 21 (*wèi shù*), and LV 13 (*zhāng mén*) are added for deficiency cold in the middle *jiao*.

DIARRHEA

Record in *Acupuncture - Moxibustion for Difficult Diseases* (*Qí Nán Zá Bìng Zhēn Jiǔ Zhì Liáo*)

Sun, female, 58, first visit was on June 8, 1988

【Chief Complaint】
Abdominal pain and diarrhea in the morning for more than 2 years

【Present Medical History】
Every morning at about 6 a.m., the patient would begin to have chills, abdominal pain, and five to six loose bowel movements; after 8 a.m., the symptoms disappeared

【Examination】
Pale tongue, with a thin white coating, thin and weak pulse

【Diagnosis】
Diarrhea (due to yang deficiency with interior cold)

【Treatment Principle】
Warm the yang to stop diarrhea

【Treatment】

ST 36 (*zú sān lǐ*)	ST 37 (*shàng jù xū*)	DU 14 (*dà zhuī*)

ST 36 (*zú sān lǐ*) and ST 37 (*shàng jù xū*) were treated with tonifying stimulation. DU 14 (*dà zhuī*) was treated for 30 minutes with moxibustion. The patient was treated once a day, with six treatments constituting one course. After two courses, the chills, abdominal pain and diarrhea were all improved; another two courses of treatment brought about a cure.

【Note】

Six o'clock in the morning is known as *Mǎo* (the fourth of the twelve Earthly Branches). During this period, yang qi arises. The *yang* qi of this patient is deficient; she has chills because it fails to arise. *Mǎo* is also the period for the qi of hand *yangming* large intestine channel to flow. As the large intestine is cold and deficient this patient has diarrhea. After *Mǎo*, her yang qi slowly rises, so the pain and diarrhea stop. ST 36 (*zú sān lǐ*) and ST 37 (*shàng jù xū*) are Lower *hé*-sea points, and are excellent in the treatment of *fu* organs. DU 14 (*dà zhuī*), the intersecting point of all yang channels, lifts and reinforces yang qi, especially with moxibustion. When the *yang* qi extends, it increases resistance to [cold] pathogens, thus her symptoms stop.

Lou Bai-ceng's Medical Record

Zhang, female, 42 years old

【Chief Complaint】

Loose stools for nearly one year

【Present Medical History】

Due to improper dietary habits, the patient began to have loose stools two to three times a day. Recently, she had symptoms of abdominal distention, fatigue, and poor appetite.

【Examination】

Sallow complexion, listlessness, tender tongue with a white coating, and a soft thready pulse

【Diagnosis】

Diarrhea (due to spleen and stomach deficiency)

【Treatment Principles】

Strengthen the spleen, harmonize the stomach, stop diarrhea

【Treatment】

BL 20 (pí shù)	ST 25 (tiān shū)	ST 36 (zú sān lǐ)

Acupuncture was performed using a lifting and thrusting tonifying method. After three treatments, the stools were firmer, after six treatments the patient's stools were completely normal. A follow-up after half a year found no recurrence.

【Note】

Her loose stools were caused by weakness of transportation and transformation functions of the spleen and stomach. Back-*shù* point, BL 20 (*pí shù*), and ST 25 (*tiān shū*), Front-*mù* point, are the places where the qi of spleen and large intestine gather. They are used together with ST 36 (*zú sān lǐ*), the *hé*-sea point of the stomach channel, to strengthen the spleen, harmonize the stomach, and regulate the qi of stomach and intestines to stop diarrhea.

Summary

Diarrhea refers to abnormal frequency and liquidity of fecal discharge, which can be seen in cases of enteritis, intestinal tuberculosis, colitis, intestinal dysfunctions, and other such illnesses. Acute cases if not resolved, can lead to chronic illness.

Main points: RN 12 (*zhōng wǎn*), ST 25 (*tiān shū*), BL 25 (*dà cháng shù*), ST 36 (*zú sān lǐ*).

DU 14 (*dà zhuī*), LI 11 (*qū chí*) and LI 4 (*hé gǔ*) are employed to treat diarrhea caused by external pathogenic factors. RN 6 (*qì hǎi*) is added if there is cold damp. ST 44 (*nèi tíng*), SP 9 (*yīn líng quán*) and LI 4 (*hé gǔ*) are used to treat damp heat presentations. LV 13 (*zhāng mén*) and SP 3 (*tài bái*) are used to treat spleen deficiency. BL 23 (*shèn shù*), DU 4 (*mìng mén*), KI 3 (*tài xī*), RN 4 (*guān yuán*), and DU 20 (*bǎi huì*) can be used to treat any associated kidney deficiency.

CONSTIPATION

Yang Jie-bin's Medical Record

Wang, male, 40, first visit was on March 17, 1964

【Chief Complaint】

Constipation for two months

【Present Medical History】

Two months ago he had diarrhea due to improper dietary habits. After being treated for the diarrhea, he ended up with constipation where he would only have a bowel movement once every three to four days; the stools were dry in the shape of sheep's feces. Other symptoms included abdominal fullness, poor appetite and clear urine.

【Examination】

Tenderness in the area of ST 25 (*tiān shū*), pale red tongue, with a thin yellow greasy coating, deep excessive pulse.

【Diagnosis】

Constipation (due to qi stagnation and intestinal dryness)

【Treatment Principles】

Open and regulate the qi of the intestines, moisten the intestines

【Treatment】

SJ 6 (*zhī gōu*)　　　　　ST 25 (*tiān shū*)　　　　　BL 25 (*dà cháng shù*)

KI 6 (*zhào hǎi*)

Treatment was given once a day with the needles retained for 30 minutes and manipulated once every three minutes. After one treatment, there was some urge to move the bowels. After three treatments, the stools became soft and discharged normally everyday in the morning. After four treatments, the bowels returned to normal.

【Note】

Constipation is usually caused by heat accumulated in the *yangming*. The intestines are dry and lacking fluids, thus causing the qi mechanism to stagnate. The treatment principle is to unobstruct the intestines by circulating the qi and moistening the intestines. ST 25 (*tiān shū*) and BL 25 (*dà cháng shù*) directly dredge the intestines. SJ 6 (*zhī gōu*), a distal point, opens the qi circulation of *sanjiao* to smooth the intestines. KI 6 (*zhào hǎi*) replenishes the kidney water and produces essence and blood to nourish yin thus moistening dryness that unblocks the dry stool.

Lou Bai-ceng's Medical Record

Du, female, 50

【Chief Complaint】

Constipation with difficulty in passing stool for two years

【Present Medical History】

She had irregular bowel movements where she would usually have one bowel movement every three to five days, or when the condition was worse, once every seven to eight days.

【Examination】

Moist tongue coating.

【Diagnosis】

Constipation (due to qi stagnation in intestines)

【Treatment Principles】

Regulate the qi mechanism, open the bowels

【Treatment】

BL 25 (dà cháng shù)	SP 15 (dà héng)	SJ 6 (zhī gōu)

Acupuncture with a draining lifting-thrusting method was given once a day. One hour after each treatment she would pass a little stool. To help with the treatment she was asked to try to have a bowel movement at a regular time in order to facilitate the formation of a new habit. After 10 treatments, her stools became normal.

【Note】

This patient was constipated due to the qi stagnation in the intestines. BL 25 (dà cháng shù) is employed to circulate qi and remove stagnation. SP 15 (dà héng) is used to promote the spleen's transportative function, thus aiding the movement of stool. SJ 6 (zhī gōu) is used to improve qi circulation of the *sanjiao*. Modern medicine holds that constipation is due to weak peristalsis. The mild lifting-thrusting method gently drains, and is used to strengthen peristalsis. If a strongly draining treatment is given, it will result in an inhibition of peristalsis.

Summary

Constipation, with difficult to pass stools which lasts for three or more days, can be due to both excess and deficiency presentations. The excess presentation refers to an obstruction of the intestines due to pathogenic factors, while in the deficient presentation it is a lack of moisture in the intestines, which causes a failure of the stool to move. Unobstructing and moistening the intestines are the treatment principles to follow.

Main points: ST 25 (tiān shū), BL 25 (dà cháng shù), ST 36 (zú sān lǐ), SJ 6 (zhī gōu).

For abdominal distention, add RN 12 (zhōng wǎn) and RN 6 (qì hǎi). For excess heat in intestines, add LI 11 (qū chí), LI 4 (hé gǔ) and BL 32 (cì liáo). For qi and blood deficiency, add BL 20 (pí shù) and BL 23 (shèn shù).

Lóng Bì (DYSURIA)

Lu Shou-yan's Medical Record

Liu, male, 51, first visit was on December 7, 1962

【Chief Complaint】

Frequent and difficult urination for more than 10 years

【Present Medical History】

In 1950 the patient fractured his lumbar vertebra. Thereafter, he had frequent urination with turbidity and loose stools

【Examination】

There was a subjective sense of throbbing below the umbilicus, the abdomen was soft, along with soreness and distention upon palpation in the region of DU 4 (*mìng mén*) and DU 3 (*yāo yáng guān*), the pulse was thin, wiry and rapid, with the proximal position being floating and weak. The pulse located at right KI 3 (*tài xī*) was deeper and weaker than that of the left side, the ST 42 (*chōng yáng*) pulse was extremely strong, and the pulse at LV 3 (*tài chōng*) was wiry and full, the patient had a flabby tongue, dirty greasy coating.

【Diagnosis】

Lóng-bì (due to deficiency complicated with excess)

【Treatment Principles】

Replenish kidney yang, reinforce the kidney and *du* vessels, clear damp heat, and unobstruct the water passages

【Treatment】

RN 3 (*zhōng jí*)	RN 6 (*qì hǎi*)	KI 10 (*yīn gǔ*)
KI 3 (*tài xī*)	BL 43 (*gāo huāng*)	ST 28 (*shuǐ dào*)

SP 6 (*sān yīn jiāo*)	DU 3 (*yāo yáng guān*)	BL 28 (*páng guāng shù*)
BL 22 (*sān jiāo shù*)	BL 39 (*wěi yáng*)	

A combination of tonifying and draining methods of lifting - thrusting was employed.

BL 39 (*wěi yáng*), BL 28 (*páng guāng shù*), SP 6 (*sān yīn jiāo*), BL 22 (*sān jiāo shù*) and ST 28 (*shuǐ dào*) were drained. The others were tonified. The needles were retained for 15 minutes. The patient was treated once a day, with 12 treatments constituting one course of treatment.

【Note】

The urinary bladder is the organ that stores urine, and with normal qi circulation urination is normal; when there are abnormalities, there will be urinary difficulty, which is known as *Lóng-bì*.

The *sanjiao* is the pathway of water, and when obstructed, urinary difficulties will appear, this is known as *Bi* - retention.

In the *Plain Questions - On the Cavity of Bone* (*Sù Wèn: Gǔ Kōng Lùn*, 素问•骨空论) is written: "*du* vessel...along the penis down...is diseased, producing difficult urination, hemorrhoid and enuresis."

This patient had damage to the *du* vessel due to the lumbar fracture, this damaged the qi, which then became deficient, resulting in poor nourishment of the lower *jiao*, impeding the qi transformation of the urinary bladder which then failed to properly discharge urine, at the same time there was a damp heat invasion; thus causing *Lóng-bì*. The weakness of the proximal pulse along with the deep and weak KI 3 (*tài xī*) pulse, points to kidney deficiency and a lack of nourishment in the lower *jiao*. Pulses that are wiry and rapid means there is heat. Turbid urination means there is damp heat falling downward.

BL 39 (*wěi yáng*), the Lower *hé*-sea of *sanjiao*, and BL 28 (*páng guāng shù*) and BL 22 (*sān jiāo shù*) where drained to clear heat from the *sanjiao* and remove damp heat in urinary bladder. ST 28 (*shuǐ dào*) and SP 6 (*sān yīn jiāo*) were also drained to induce diuresis.

Tonification treatment was used on KI 10 (*yīn gǔ*), the *hé*-sea water point of the foot *shaoyin* kidney channel, KI 3 (*tài xī*), *yuán*-source point of the kidney, and BL 43 (*gāo huāng*), the point from which the foot *shaoyin* kidney channel enters into the kidney itself and which also connects with the urinary bladder. RN 6 (*qì hǎi*), the sea of *yuán*-source primordial qi, was also tonified to replenish kidney yang. Additionally, DU 3 (*yāo yáng guān*) was selected to tonify yang of *du* vessel and RN 3 (*zhōng jí*), Front-*mù* of the urinary bladder, was treated with tonifying methods to strengthen its ability to transform bladder qi.

This patient's condition is one of deficiency complicated by excess. Therefore, reducing the Back-*shù* points decreases the pathogenic heat in the urinary bladder; tonifying the Front-*mù* points promotes kidney yang. This treatment method can be considered to be one where there is draining with tonification.

Yang Yong-xuan's Medical Record

Wang, male, 20

【Chief Complaint】
Retention of urine for two days

【Present Medical History】
This patient is mentally ill and sustained a severe injury to his left foot by jumping off a building, which lead to an amputation. After the operation, he suffered from urinary retention and abdominal distention.

【Examination】
Distal and middle pulse strong, proximal pulse was thin

【Diagnosis】
Bì - retention of urine (due to upper excess and lower deficiency)

【Treatment Principles】
Drain the excess, tonify the deficiency

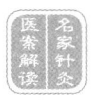

【Treatment】

LI 6 (*piān lì*)	LU 7 (*liè quē*)	
Right side:	LV 8 (*qū quán*)	SP 9 (*yīn líng quán*)
	KI 3 (*tài xī*)	

A combination of tonifying and draining methods of rapid and slow insertion and withdrawal of the needle was employed. KI 3 (*tài xī*) was tonified and the other points were drained. Three hours after the treatment, the urination was smooth. More treatments were given to consolidate the effect.

【Note】

Plain Questions - Expounding on the Energies of Five Viscera (*Sù Wèn: Xuān Míng Wǔ Qì*, 素问·宣明五气) says: "The urinary bladder is disordered, causing *Lóng* - dysuria." Dysfunctions of lower *jiao* qi transformation or an accumulation of dampness and heat block the channels and collaterals which leads to a disruption of the function in the urinary bladder; this is usually an excess presentation. In this case the patient's retention of urine with fullness in the lower abdomen is due to the failure of qi in the pelvis to go downward. The sudden onset of his urinary retention is due to heat. His pulse reflects excess in the upper *jiao* and deficiency in the lower. Professor Yang treated him by draining the *taiyin* and *jueyin* channels and tonifying the *shaoyin* to smooth the qi, thus allowing the urine to pass without difficulty.

Cao Huai-ren's Medical Record

Zhang, male, 28

【Chief Complaint】

Dysuria for two days and dribbling scanty urination for one day

【Present Medical History】

Ten days before his visit the patient had the common cold for 10 days and began to experience difficulties in passing urine. Only 40ml urine was discharged in eight hours, then it completely stopped. He had an insufferable distending pain in his lower abdomen, sweating and frigid extremities.

【Examination】

The urinary bladder was full

【Diagnosis】

Bì - retention of urine (due to external pathogenic factors inhibiting the diffusion of lung qi)

【Treatment Principles】

Diffuse the lung, regulate the lower *jiao*

【Treatment】

LU 7 (*liè quē*)	LU 9 (*tài yuān*)	RN 4 (*guān yuán*)
KI 6 (*zhào hǎi*)		

LU 7 (*liè quē*) and LU 9 (*tài yuān*) were needled with the needles being retained for 10 minutes. RN 4 (*guān yuán*) and KI 6 (*zhào hǎi*) were needled with strong stimulation and then immediatly removed. About 10 minutes later, the patient was able to urinate and the pain stopped.

【Note】

In this case urinary retention comes along with the common cold due to the lung's ability to diffuse downward being obstructed by external pathogens, thus blocking the water pathways, resulting in not a single drop of urine being expelled.

LU 9 (*tài yuān*), *yuán*-source point of lung channel, LU 7 (*liè quē*) and KI 6 (*zhào hǎi*) are the confluent points of their respective extraordinary channels, they all function to disperse lung qi. RN 4 (*guān yuán*) is the intersection point of the *ren* vessel with the three foot yin channels; it is an important point for treating urinary retention. As stated in the *Experience on*

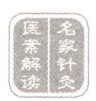

Acupuncture and Moxibustion Therapy (Zhēn Jiǔ Zī Shēng Jīng, 针灸资生经): "The point RN 4 (*guān yuán*) is indicated in diseases with urine retention." When combined with KI 6 (*zhào hǎi*) it helps to promote qi transformation in the lower *jiao*.

Summary

Lóng Bì (癃闭) is a condition where it is either difficult to expel urine, the stream of urine is weak, even to the point of complete retention of urine without the ability to expel even a drop. This condition can be caused by either damp heat in the lower *jiao*, kidney yang deficiency or injury due to trauma.

Main points: RN 3 (*zhōng jí*), SP 6 (*sān yīn jiāo*), BL 32 (*cì liáo*).

Associated points:

SP 9 (*yīn líng quán*) and BL 28 (*páng guāng shù*) are used to treat heat in the lower *jiao*. BL 23 (*shèn shù*) and RN 4 (*guān yuán*) are used with moxibustion to tonify kidney yang. BL 22 (*sān jiāo shù*) and RN 6 (*qì hǎi*) are used for injury due to trauma.

In the treatment of *Bì* - retention of urine, if the routine points are not effective, LV 10 (*zú wǔ lǐ*) can be added as it is a point on the foot *jueyin* liver channel which "goes along the medial aspect of thigh, enters into the perineum, curves around the genitals and arrives in the lower abdomen."

Lìn Zhèng (STRANGURIA)

Yang Jia-san's Medical Record

X X, male, 71, first visit was on August 26, 1996

【Chief Complaint】

Frequent urination

【Present Medical History】

The patient needed to urinate once every hour in the daytime and six to seven times at night, he had accompanying symptoms of distending pain in the lower abdomen, and was diagnosed with benign prostate hypertrophy. Treatment with western medicine did not produce any significant results. He was referred for an operation, which he refused as he had a pacemaker, so came for acupuncture.

【Examination】

Tongue normal, with a thin white coating, pulse was deep and thin

【Diagnosis】

Lìn Zhèng - stranguria (due to qi *Lìn* deficiency syndrome)

【Treatment Principles】

Tonify *yuán*-source qi, regulate the qi mechanism

【Treatment】

LU 7 (*liè quē*)	KI 6 (*zhào hǎi*)	SP 6 (*sān yīn jiāo*)

Treatment was given once every other day using medium stimulation, which reduced the frequency to twice a night. After ten treatments his urination returned to normal.

Two weeks later, the patient returned complaining that one week after his last course of acupuncture he was getting up four to five times a night to urinate. He also had headache, dizziness, fatigue, and a poor appetite.

【Treatment】

Previous points plus:		
GB 20 (*fēng chí*)	DU 20 (*bǎi huì*)	LI 4 (*hé gǔ*)

After treatment the patient urinated two to three times a night; his headache and dizziness disappeared. He was treated every other day for a month, during this time he usually would urinate once or twice a night, occasionally three times. He continued to have some lower abdominal discomfort. A three month follow up found that his condition had been stabilized.

【Note】

Benign prostate hypertrophy is a common disease seen in middle aged and elderly men. In mild cases it manifests with symptoms of frequent urination and a weak stream, in more serious cases there is urinary retention; this falls into the categories of *Lìn Zhèng* - stranguria and *Lóng Bì* - dysuria in traditional Chinese medicine. The causative factors are kidney qi deficiency, difficulties with qi transformation in the *sanjiao*, failure of the urinary bladder to properly open and close, retained dampness which creates stagnation transforming into heat, and damp heat clumping in the lower *jiao*; these are complicated patterns which are a mixture of both excess and deficiency. Professor Yang holds that the treatment should be aimed at tonifying *yuán*-source qi and regulating qi mechanism of the *sanjiao*. The basic point pair is LU 7 (*liè quē*) and KI 6 (*zhào hǎi*). LU 7 (*liè quē*) is both a *luò*-connecting point and the confluent point, which opens to the *ren* vessel; it diffuses lung qi to open the water passages and it functions to tonify and regulate kidney qi. It is essential in cases of "frequent, but scanty urination". KI 6 (*zhào hǎi*) regulates and tonifies kidney qi, which in turn promotes the qi transformation of the urinary bladder. For cases where there is a significant deficiency, SP 6 (*sān yīn jiāo*), BL 23 (*shèn shù*) and BL 28 (*páng guāng shù*) should be used to tonify kidney qi. For significant signs of damp heat, which are accompanied by painful urination, SI 5 (*yáng gǔ*) and RN 4 (*guān yuán*) are used to clear heat and drain dampness.

EDEMA

Lu Shou-yan's Medical Record

Xu, female, 54

【Chief Complaint】

Edema of the whole body

【Present Medical History】

The patient's edema started in the lower limbs and gradually included the abdominal region and face. She was listless with cold limbs, had abdominal fullness, poor appetite, loose stools, and scanty urination.

【Examination】

Pale swollen tongue, with a moist, white coating, pulse was deep and thin

【Diagnosis】

Edema (due to spleen and kidney yang deficiency)

【Treatment Principles】

Warm the yang to strengthen the spleen, circulate qi to induce diuresis

【Treatment】

BL 13 (fèi shù)	BL 20 (pí shù)	BL 23 (shèn shù)
RN 6 (qì hǎi)	RN 9 (shuǐ fēn)	

Moxibustion was applied to RN 9 (shuǐ fēn) for 5~10 minutes. The other points were also tonified. Warming needle moxibustion was applied to BL 20 (pí shù) and BL 23 (shèn shù) after the needles had been manipulated with a lifting-thrusting and rotating motion. RN 6 (qì hǎi) was needled with a lifting-thrusting motion, but not retained.

On the second visit, her edema was reduced by half along with an increase in urine output; she still had loose stools, and a pale tongue with white coating, the pulse still was deep and thin. The above-mentioned points plus SP 9 (yīn líng quán) were treated. SP 9 (yīn líng quán) was first tonified with warming needle moxibustion and then drained.

On the third visit, her edema was almost completely gone. Her appetite improved and she felt energetic. There was no more abdominal distention. Urination and bowel movements had returned to normal. The tongue was slightly pale, with a thin white coating. To warm the yang, strengthen the spleen and consolidate the treatment, BL 20 (pí shù), BL 23 (shèn shù), RN 6 (qì hǎi) and ST 36 (zú sān lǐ) were all tonified. BL 20 (pí shù) and BL 23 (shèn shù)

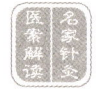

were needled briefly and without retention the needles, warming needle moxibustion was applied on all other points.

【Note】

This patient manifests yin edema caused by spleen and kidney yang deficiency. Professor Lu selected BL 13 (*fèi shù*) to diffuse the lung qi, BL 20 (*pí shù*) to strengthen the spleen to control water, BL 23 (*shèn shù*) to reinforce kidney to warm yang, RN 6 (*qì hǎi*) to replenish genuine *yuán*-source, and applied moxibustion to RN 9 (*shuǐ fēn*) to induce diuresis to relieve the edema. On the second visit, SP 9 (*yīn líng quán*), the water point of the earth channel, was tonified to strengthen the earth, and drained to control the water. Professor Lu's simultaneous usage of draining while tonifying brings about wondrous effect in promoting urination to get rid of edema. On the third visit, the pathogenic factors were already mostly gone, but the normal qi was weak; strengthening the earth to control water was the right principle to follow to successfully resolve this patient's edema.

Zheng Yi-zhong's Medical Record

Ren, female, 21, first visit was on February 9, 1960

【Chief Complaint】

Facial edema and swollen feet, recurrent lumbar pain

【Present Medical History】

Half a year ago the patient was admitted into the hospital for pyelitis and discharged when improved. Afterwards she had repeated occurrences of edema, especially when exposed to cold. Today she presented with a puffy face and edema in her feet, lumbar pain and frequent and urgent urination

【Examination】

Urine: protein (+), WBC (+), platycyte (+), RBC 1~4. Pale red tongue with a thin white coating, deep and a slightly slow pulse

【Diagnosis】

Edema (due to kidney qi deficiency)

【Treatment Principles】

Warm and tonify the *mingmen*

【Treatment】

Moxibustion:	BL 23 (*shèn shù*)

Moxibustion was applied to BL 23 (*shèn shù*) once a day; 30 minutes each time. After one treatment, the edema was significantly improved. After 10 treatments, the symptoms disappeared and urination became normal. A one year follow-up showed no recurrence.

【Note】

The prolonged illness of this patient lead to kidney qi deficiency, with a weakness of the *mingmen* fire, producing a condition of deficiency cold which effected the water metabolism. Moxibustion to BL 23 (*shèn shù*) is very effective in warming and tonifying the *mingmen*, which activates the urinary bladder and promotes diuresis; thus treating edema.

Summary

Edema is attributed to weakness of the lung, spleen and kidney, so that water is out of control, thus running abnormally to the skin. Yin and yang, exterior and interior, deficiency and excess should be clearly differentiated for setting up treatment principles.

Invasion of wind damp is usually a sign of yang edema, characterized by its quick onset from face and head to the whole body. Internal factors usually induce yin edema which is often due to yang qi deficiency characterized by a slow onset from feet or eyelids and then progressing gradually to the entire body.

Main points for yang edema:

LI 4 (*hé gǔ*), LI 11 (*qū chí*), LU 7 (*liè quē*), BL 13 (*fèi shù*).

Main points for yin edema:

BL 20 (*pí shù*), BL 23 (*shèn shù*), RN 6 (*qì hǎi*), RN 9 (*shuǐ fēn*), SP 9 (*yīn líng quán*).

DU 26 (*rén zhōng*) is useful for facial edema. LI 6 (*piān lì*) treats edema in the upper limbs. SP 6 (*sān yīn jiāo*) and GB 41 (*zú lín qì*) treat the lower limbs, for these lower points in the legs, especially for serious or prolonged cases, thick needles are used to help promote water metabolism.

Xiāo Kě (DIABETES)

Wang Fa-xiang's Medical Record

Zhao, female, 49, first visit on March 7, 1995

【Chief Complaint】
Pain in the lower limbs for three weeks

【Present Medical History】
The patient suffered from diabetes for three years. She currently had symptoms, which included a dry month, thirst, fatigue, irritability, dizziness and tinnitus.

【Examination】
Fasting blood-glucose 14 mmol/L, glucose in urine (+++), dark tongue, thin pulse

【Diagnosis】
Xiāo Kě - diabetes (due to qi yin deficiency, obstruction of channels)

【Treatment Principles】
Benefit the qi, nourish the yin, invigorate the blood and open the collaterals

【Treatment】

BL 20 (*pí shù*)	BL 23 (*shèn shù*)	BL 40 (*wěi zhōng*)

ST 36 (*zú sān lǐ*)	BL 57 (*chéng shān*)	SP 6 (*sān yīn jiāo*)
KI 3 (*tài xī*)	KI 2 (*rán gǔ*)	

The patient must experience the sensation of "de qi" for this treatment to be effective. Tonify ST 36 (*zú sān lǐ*), and use an even method on the other points. Treatment should be given once a day, with 15 treatments constituting one course. After one course of treatment, this patient's pain and thirst were greatly reduced, and fasting blood-glucose fell to 8 mmol/L. With another course of treatment, her pain and all the other symptoms disappeared. A follow-up found her condition to be stable.

【Note】

The pain in the lower extremities caused by *Xiāo Kě* - diabetes is due to hypofunction of the *zang-fu* organs resulting in a deficiency of qi, blood and body fluids, this insufficiency leads to poor nourishment of the limbs. This condition is primarily one of deficiency, but complicated by the excess of stasis. The lower limb pain in this patient is related to her diabetes. Therefore, the treatment should be focused on the spleen and kidney. As *The Great Compendium of Acupuncture and Moxibustion* (*Zhēn Jiǔ Dà Chéng*, 针灸大成) summarized: *Xiāo Kě* is due to "exhaustion of kidney water, disharmony between water and fire, and dysfunction of both the spleen and kidney."

BL 20 (*pí shù*), BL 23 (*shèn shù*), ST 36 (*zú sān lǐ*), SP 6 (*sān yīn jiāo*), KI 3 (*tài xī*) and KI 2 (*rán gǔ*) are used to treat the root of this patient's illness; BL 57 (*chéng shān*) and BL 40 (*wěi zhōng*) are added to relieve the resulting symptom pain.

Summary

Xiāo Kě (消渴), diabetes in modern medicine, relates to upper, middle and lower *jiao*, and all five *zang* organs, especially spleen and kidney. This disease can be seen to have three stages. In the initial stage, the pathological condition is one of heat that exhausts body fluid; thus manifesting as yin deficiency and dry heat, with symptoms such as thirst and ravenous appetite. Due to the depletion of body fluids there is a flaring of the stomach fire. Additionally, there is an accompanying deficiency of the spleen and kidney. The high sugar level of the urine is due to spleen deficiency resulting in incomplete absorption of the food essence, which then falls down into the bladder. The increased volume of urine is the outcome of kidney qi failing to control the water. In the middle stage yin deficiency leads to qi exhaustion. Therefore, signs of qi and yin exhaustion are both to be found. At the same time, signs of stasis appear due to the inability of qi to circulate the blood. Weakness of the *zang-fu* lead to a variety of complications and dysfunctions that are more severe as time goes on. In the late stage, the deficiency qi and yin become more severe and blood stasis aggravates the situation, thus are seen the manifestations of both yin and yang deficiency as more organs become diseased. This is why diabetes in the late stage is always complicated by the development of multiple pathologies.

The treatment principles vary depending on the individual condition of the patient; which can include clearing of heat, moistening of dryness, tonification of qi, nourishment of the yin, strengthening of the kidney to consolidate the root, invigorating the blood, opening the collaterals, and cooling blood and promoting its circulation.

Points: Front: KI 2 (*rán gǔ*), KI 3 (*tài xī*), SP 6 (*sān yīn jiāo*), ST 36 (*zú sān lǐ*), PC 6 (*nèi guān*). Back: BL 20 (*pí shù*), BL 23 (*shèn shù*), BL 17 (*gé shù*).

LU 10 (*yú jì*) is added for thirst. ST 44 (*nèi tíng*) is used to treat voracious appetite. RN 4 (*guān yuán*) is used for polyuria. BL 40 (*wěi zhōng*), BL 57 (*chéng shān*), and BL 60 (*kūn lún*) needled through to KI 3 (*tài xī*) treats pain or numbness of the lower limbs. LV 3 (*tài chōng*) and ST 9 (*rén yíng*) treat hypertension. ST 25 (*tiān shū*), SJ 6 (*zhī gōu*) and ST 40 (*fēng lóng*) are needled for constipation. ST 25 (*tiān shū*), ST 37 (*shàng jù xū*) and ST 39 (*xià jù xū*) can be added for diarrhea. BL 1 (*jīng míng*) and LV 3 (*tài chōng*) are points for treating problems with the eyes. HT 7 (*shén mén*) and PC 6 (*nèi guān*) treat palpitations. HT 7 (*shén mén*) and SP 6 (*sān yīn jiāo*) can be added for insomnia. RN 12 (*zhōng wǎn*) and PC 6 (*nèi guān*) treat fullness in the chest. RN 17 (*dàn zhōng*) and PC 6 (*nèi guān*) are used for chest pain. LI 4 (*hé gǔ*) and KI 7 (*fù liū*) help to control sweating. SI 3 (*hòu xī*) and HT 6 (*yīn xì*) are used in particular for night sweating. LI 11 (*qū chí*) and SP 10 (*xuè hǎi*) treat itching. LV 5 (*lí gōu*) is for perineal itching. KI 12 (*dà hè*), RN 4 (*guān yuán*) and LV 3 (*tài chōng*) can treat impotence; and moxibustion at RN 4 (*guān yuán*) and RN 8 (*shén què*) treats deficiency cold.

PALPITATIONS

Lu Shou-yan's Medical Record

Li, male, 50

【Chief Complaint】

Palpitations

【Present Medical History】

This patient's palpitations began after an extended period of feeling depressed due to having some kind of setback at work. The palpitations come and go, and he had a sense of fear which interfered with his sleep.

【Examination】

Flushed face, proximal pulse was thin and weak, distal pulse beating hard

【Diagnosis】

Palpitations (due to phlegm fire disturbing heart)

【Treatment Principles】

Expand the chest, relieve depression, transform phlegm, calm the mind

【Treatment】

BL 15 (*xīn shù*)	RN 14 (*jù quē*)	RN 4 (*guān yuán*)
PC 6 (*nèi guān*)	ST 40 (*fēng lóng*)	LV 2 (*xíng jiān*)

Tonifying-draining was done by means of lifting-thrusting. RN 4 (*guān yuán*) was tonified, PC 6 (*nèi guān*) was first drained and then manipulated to circulate the qi of the chest. BL 15 (*xīn shù*) first drained and then tonified (See the note below for an explanation of the Yang *Hidden within* Yin *Method* - [*Yīn Zhōng Yǐn Yáng*, 阴中隐阳法] technique), all the other points were drained.

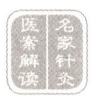

After three treatments the palpitations were significantly reduced and his sense of fear abated. Another month of acupuncture was given to consolidate the treatment.

【Note】

According to *The Yellow Emperor's Internal Classic* (*Huáng Dì Nèi Jīng*, 黄帝内经) "over thinking and dissatisfaction" are causes of depression. If this continues over a prolonged period of time it will transform into fire, produce phlegm and consume the yin and blood. The phlegm is stirred up by fire which then disturbs the heart. In that the blood fails to nourish the heart, and the mind which is stored in the heart loses its abode, symptoms of palpitations with fear and poor sleep arise. This patient is suffering from phlegm fire, which developed from qi stagnation, that disturbs the mind which is stored in the heart. Professor Lu uses PC 6 (*nèi guān*) and RN 14 (*jù quē*) to expand the chest, relieve depression and calm the mind. LV 2 (*xíng jiān*) is drained to calm the liver thereby eliminating qi stagnation. PC 6 (*nèi guān*) is drained to quickly circulate qi of the chest. BL 15 (*xīn shù*) is first drained to remove fire and tonified to firm the deficient yang, Lu uses a particular method, which he describes as **Drain First, Then Reinforce** (Yin *Zhōng Yǐn* Yang). RN 4 (*guān yuán*) is tonified to replenish essence which nourishes the heart. ST 40 (*fēng lóng*) is drained to bring down turbid phlegm and stop it from disturbing the heart. In this way with three treatments the palpitations are greatly reduced and within one month the patient was cured.

> *Yang Hidden within Yin Method* (*Yīn Zhōng Yǐn Yáng* 阴中隐阳法)*:*
>
> *This method involves manipulating the needle at both deep and shallow levels in the following way:*
>
> *The needle is inserted first to the deep level, then manipulated to drain with six quick lifting and then slow inserting thrusts; the needle is then lifted to the shallow level and manipulated to tonify with nine quick thrusting and slow lifting motions. It is used to treat illness which first manifest with heat and then turn to cold.*
>
> *This technique is the opposite of the Yin Hidden within Yang Method (Yáng Zhōng Yǐn Yīn, 阳中隐阴法). Both of them are indicated for use in complicated syndromes with simultaneous presentations of deficiency and excess.*

Cheng Xin-nong's Medical Record

Wu, female, 48, first visit was on May 11, 1992

【Chief Complaint】

Palpitations with shortness of breath for four years

【Present Medical History】

At the beginning of her illness the patient went to a hospital in Beijing for an examination, she was not found to have any problems with any of her organs. She had symptoms of heart palpitations, shortness of breath, insomnia and forgetfulness; she experienced dizziness, tinnitus, a sore back, dry stools, and scanty irregular periods, which were dark in color and contained clots.

【Examination】

Lustreless complexion, red tongue, thin contracted tongue and with cracks and a white coating, the pulse was deep, thin and wiry.

【Diagnosis】

Palpitations (due to yin deficiency with fire)

【Treatment Principles】

Moisten yin to reduce fire, calm the heart and mind

【Treatment】

RN 14 (jù quē)	RN 17 (dàn zhōng)	BL 15 (xīn shù)
BL 23 (shèn shù)	PC 7 (dà líng)	PC 6 (nèi guān)
HT 7 (shén mén)	SP 6 (sān yīn jiāo)	KI 3 (tài xī)
LV 3 (tài chōng)		

BL 15 (xīn shù) and BL 23 (shèn shù) were treated with quick needling. SP 6 (sān yīn jiāo) and KI 3 (tài xī) where needled with a tonifying method; other points were treated with an even method.

After one course of treatment the patient's palpitations and shortness of breath were reduced. She was given two more courses of treatment, although not in succession, to consolidate her condition, which stabilized with only occasional palpitations.

【Note】

Blood deficiency leads to the rise of deficient fire, disturbing the mind stored in the heart and leading to palpitations, shortness of breath and insomnia. BL 15 (*xīn shù*), the Back-*shù* of the heart, RN 14 (*jù quē*), the Front-*mù* of the heart, PC 6 (*nèi guān*), the *luò*-connecting point, and RN 17 (*dàn zhōng*) the influential point of qi, function together to tonify qi thus producing blood which nourishes the heart, thus stopping palpitations. The other points reduce fire through the moistening of yin and settle the heart and calm the mind.

Summary

Palpitations, known as *Jīng Jì* (惊悸) in Chinese medicine, are treated using a combination of Back-*shù* and Front-*mù* points.

Commonly used points: BL 15 (*xīn shù*), RN 14 (*jù quē*), HT 7 (*shén mén*), PC 6 (*nèi guān*).

For those who have heart blood deficiency, add BL 20 (*pí shù*) and BL 21 (*wèi shù*) to promote blood production; for yin deficiency with fire, add BL 18 (*gān shù*), KI 3 (*tài xī*), BL 23 (*shèn shù*) and LV 3 (*tài chōng*) to replenish yin to smooth the liver and improve communication between the heart and kidney; for yang deficiency with dampness, add RN 4 (*guān yuán*), RN 17 (*dàn zhōng*) and ST 36 (*zú sān lǐ*) to strengthen the spleen to transform fluids; for sudden fright, add *sì shén cōng* (EX-HN1) and *yìn táng* (EX-HN3) to settle and calm the mind.

Bú Mèi (INSOMNIA)

Lu Shou-yan's Medical Record

Li, male, 33

【Chief Complaint】

Difficulties in falling asleep for half a year

【Present Medical History】

This patient had occasional difficulties with falling asleep; lately his sleep problem had became worse. Additionally he had dizziness, tinnitus, dry throat, irritability, seminal emissions and lumbar soreness.

【Examination】

Red tongue with a sparse coating, and a thin rapid pulse

【Diagnosis】

Insomnia (due to disharmony between heart and kidney)

【Treatment Principles】

Strengthen water to control fire, facilitate communication between the heart and kidney

【Treatment】

BL 15 (*xīn shù*)	BL 23 (*shèn shù*)	HT 7 (*shén mén*)
SP 6 (*sān yīn jiāo*)		

Moxibustion with 3 grain-sized cones was done at BL 15 (*xīn shù*). Lifting-thrusting needling without retention of needles was done at the other points. BL 23 (*shèn shù*) and SP 6 (*sān yīn jiāo*) were tonified. HT 7 (*shén mén*) was drained.

Second visit: His condition was improved, red tongue, thin pulse.

【Treatment】

BL 14 (*jué yīn shù*)	BL 23 (*shèn shù*)	HT 7 (*shén mén*)
SP 6 (*sān yīn jiāo*)	KI 3 (*tài xī*)	PC 6 (*nèi guān*)

Moxibustion with 3 grain-sized cones was done at BL 14 (*jué yīn shù*). Lifting-thrusting needling without retention of the needles was done at the other points. BL 23 (*shèn shù*), SP 6 (*sān yīn jiāo*) and KI 3 (*tài xī*) were

tonified. HT 7 (*shén mén*) and PC 6 (*nèi guān*) were drained.

Third visit: The patient could sleep soundly and his spirit felt much stronger. The dizziness, tinnitus, dry throat and irritability disappeared. He still had a red tongue, with a sparse coating, and a thin pulse. The treatment principles were still to facilitate communication between the heart and kidney, accompanied by tonifying and harmonizing the spleen and stomach to produce blood to calm the mind.

【Treatment】

PC 6 (*nèi guān*)	HT 7 (*shén mén*)	SP 6 (*sān yīn jiāo*)
BL 20 (*pí shù*)	ST 36 (*zú sān lǐ*)	KI 3 (*tài xī*)

Lifting-thrusting needling without retention of the needles was done. PC 6 (*nèi guān*) and HT 7 (*shén mén*) were drained. Other points were tonified.

【Note】

The heart is the house of mind and kidney the house of essence. Dizziness, tinnitus, seminal emissions and lumbar soreness are all signs of a deficiency of kidney essence; dry throat and irritability are indicative of yin deficiency with fire; a red tongue and rapid pulse point to the flaring of fire. Professor Lu treated this patient with the intent of strengthening water to control fire, and to facilitate communication between the heart and kidney. Moxibustion with 3 cones done at BL 15 (*xīn shù*) was to drive out the fire. HT 7 (*shén mén*) was drained to clear heart fire and settle the mind. Tonification of BL 23 (*shèn shù*) and SP 6 (*sān yīn jiāo*) was to strengthen water and control fire.

On the second visit, moxibustion with 3 cones at BL 14 (*jué yīn shù*) was employed to reduce heart fire, PC 6 (*nèi guān*) was drained to settle the mind, and KI 3 (*tài xī*) was tonified to replenish water. On the third visit, moxibustion was not used, but BL 20 (*pí shù*) and ST 36 (*zú sān lǐ*) were added to strengthen spleen and stomach, thus producing blood to calm the mind. Three treatments successfully cured this patient's half year of insomnia.

Xiao Shao-qing's Medical Record

Li, female, 67, first visit was on October 24, 1994

【Chief Complaint】

Insomnia for more than 30 years, worse in the past year

【Present Medical History】

One year ago, the patient's insomnia became worse after the death of her husband. She could not sleep without taking medication. In 1992 after a cholecystectomy she began to have indigestion with diarrhea. At the time of her visit she had difficulties with falling asleep, and when she did sleep she had nightmares. She was dizzy and was in a low mood. She had a tendency to over-think, was anxious and had a poor appetite; her stools were also loose.

【Previous medical history】

Cholelithiasis. Cholecystectomy 2 years previously

【Examination】

Pale tongue, white greasy coating, wiry and slippery pulse

【Diagnosis】

Insomnia (due to phlegm retention with qi stagnation, restlessness of mind)

【Treatment Principles】

Transform phlegm, relieve stagnation, settle the heart, calm the mind

【Treatment】

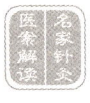

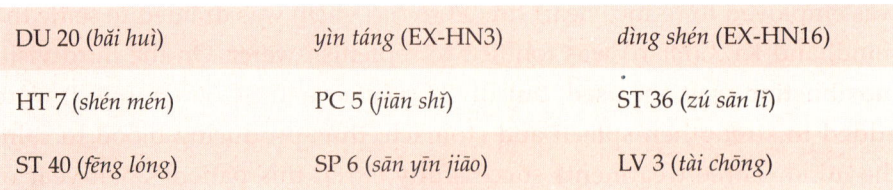

DU 20 (*bǎi huì*)	*yìn táng* (EX-HN3)	*dìng shén* (EX-HN16)
HT 7 (*shén mén*)	PC 5 (*jiān shǐ*)	ST 36 (*zú sān lǐ*)
ST 40 (*fēng lóng*)	SP 6 (*sān yīn jiāo*)	LV 3 (*tài chōng*)

An even method was applied; the needles were retained for 20 minutes and manipulated every 10 minutes. Treatment was given once a day.

On the second visit she said that she felt good after the previous treatment, but still did not sleep well. The same treatment was given to her. On the third visit, she said she slept for five hours without taking medication. After one course of treatment, she could sleep about 10 hours. The nightmares stopped, her appetite improved, her pulse was a bit slow but forceful and her tongue and coating tended toward normal.

【Note】

This patient generally is prone to overthinking, this easily leads to constraint of the liver qi. Add in the additional stress in her life and the stagnated liver qi is made worse, which then in turn attacks the middle *jiao*. Furthermore, the cholecystectomy damaged the qi of the middle *jiao*, hence the spleen and stomach are weak, and the production of phlegm is the result. The stagnated liver qi and phlegm disturb the heart, causing restlessness of mind, thus poor sleep. Professor Xiao used *yìn táng* (EX-HN3) and *dìng shén* (EX-HN16) in combination with DU 20 (*bǎi huì*) to open the *du* vessel to wake up the mind. HT 7 (*shén mén*) and PC 5 (*jiān shǐ*) were used to calm the mind and benefit consciousness. ST 36 (*zú sān lǐ*), SP 6 (*sān yīn jiāo*) and ST 40 (*fēng lóng*) are used to strengthen the spleen which in turn benefit dampness and transform phlegm. LV 3 (*tài chōng*) was treated to calm the the liver and regulate the qi. The success of this treatment is due to the principle of transforming phlegm, regulating stagnated qi, and settling the mind and calming the heart.

Dìng shén (EX-HN16) is located at the conjunction of the lower and middle 1/3 of the philtrum. Pinch the skin, and insert a 3 inch filiform needle horizontally about 2.5 inch at an angle of 15° to the subcutaneous level. It produces very strong sensations of soreness and distention. After a while, the patient will feel relaxed and may even fall asleep. This is an experiential point that Professor Xiao uses to treat insomnia with irritability. He also uses it to treat mental disorders such as epilepsy, and gets good result too.

Cheng Xin-nong's Medical Record

Wu, male, 59, first visit was on September 12, 1992

【Chief Complaint】

Poor sleep over 30 years

【Present Medical History】

In the past three years, the patient could not sleep at all without the aid of a sleeping pill, he was completely dependent on them. Two years ago he went to a Beijing hospital to have his liver function tested, his blood test showed a higher than normal level of bilirubin and he was diagnosed with gastrointestinal dysfunction. At this time, he had difficulties in falling asleep, along with dream-disturbed sleep; especially when tired, he could not sleep at all. Additionally, he had abdominal distention, poor appetite, diarrhea after drinking milk, soreness in lumbar region, frequent flatulence, and bowel movements two to three times a day.

【Examination】

Patient's tongue was pale purple, with a tip red and white coating; wiry pulse

【Diagnosis】

Insomnia (due to disharmony between spleen and stomach)

【Treatment Principles】

Strengthen the spleen, harmonize the stomach, settle the heart and calm the mind

【Treatment】

RN 12 (zhōng wǎn)	ST 25 (tiān shū)	RN 6 (qì hǎi)
PC 6 (nèi guān)	HT 7 (shén mén)	ST 36 (zú sān lǐ)
SP 6 (sān yīn jiāo)	KI 3 (tài xī)	

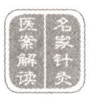

RN 6 (*qì hǎi*) and ST 36 (*zú sān lǐ*) were tonified; the other points were treated with an even method.

After four courses of treatment, his spleen and stomach functions gradually improved, his sleep was better and the dosage of the sleep medication was reduced by half. Another four courses of treatment, although intermittent, helped him to sleep six to eight hours each night without the need for medication.

【Note】

The spleen oversees transport and transformation of food essence and sends the clear essential substance upward to nourish. When this function has been weakened, the heart will lack nourishment. The stomach receives food and sends the roughly digested food downward. When the stomach qi is disharmonious it goes up instead of down, this upward movement will disturb the spirit [stored in the heart]; thus insomnia. *sea of qi*

Stomach RN 12 (*zhōng wǎn*), ST 25 (*tiān shū*), RN 6 (*qì hǎi*) and ST 36 (*zú sān lǐ*) are selected to promote the spleen in its transportive and transformation function, harmonize the stomach in digestion and get rid of distention. PC 6 (*nèi guān*), HT 7 (*shén mén*) and SP 6 (*sān yīn jiāo*) are experiential points for treating insomnia. PC 6 (*nèi guān*) is the *luò*-connecting, HT 7 (*shén mén*) is the *yuán*-source, and SP 6 (*sān yīn jiāo*) is the intersection point of spleen, liver and kidney channels, they settle the heart and calm the mind. KI 3 (*tài xī*) and HT 7 (*shén mén*) open communication between the heart and kidney.

Summary

Bú Mèi (不寐) is modern medicine's name for insomnia. "When yang enters into yin, one sleeps. When yang comes out of yin, one wakes up." Zhang Jingyue says: "Sleep depends on yin that nourishes the mind. When the mind rests well, one sleeps well. When the mind is restless, one cannot sleep well." Problems with sleep can be due to restlessness of mind which is the result of external pathological factors or it can be due to internal causes such a deficiency of the nourishing qi. Heart and spleen deficiency, yin deficiency with fire, liver and gall bladder fire or disharmony of the stomach are all common causes of insomnia. The treatment principles are to settle the heart and calm the mind. The stimulation of acupuncture points should not be strong, thus avoiding disturbing the mind.

Main Points: HT 7 (*shén mén*), PC 6 (*nèi guān*), SP 6 (*sān yīn jiāo*).

BL 15 (*xīn shù*) and BL 20 (*pí shù*) are added for heart and spleen deficiency. BL 15 (*xīn shù*), BL 23 (*shèn shù*), KI 3 (*tài xī*) are used to treat yin deficiency with fire. Other points such as KI 6 (*zhào hǎi*) can be used to regulate the *qiao mai*. BL 18 (*gān shù*), BL 19 (*dǎn shù*), LV 2 (*xíng jiān*), GB 12 (*wán gǔ*) are used to treat liver and gall bladder fire; BL 21 (*wèi shù*), RN 12 (*zhōng wǎn*), ST 36 (*zú sān lǐ*) are added for disharmony of the stomach.

HEADACHE

Cheng Xin-nong's Medical Record

Li, male, 52, first visit was on November 22, 1985

【Chief Complaint】
Paroxysmal headache at the right side for four days

【Present Medical History】
The patient recounts that he began to have this headache during a period when he was very busy at work. The top and right side of head would be intensely painful, it would come on with a sudden violent pain, as if he suddenly had bashed his head against a wall. The pain was unendurable and lasted just a few seconds with an interval of 10-30 minutes between each occurrence. There were accompanying symptoms of dizziness, palpitations, poor sleep, a bitter taste in mouth, he was short-tempered, irritable and had dry stools.

【Examination】
The sides and tip of the tongue were red, with a yellow coating in the middle, his pulse was wiry.

【Diagnosis】

Headache (due to liver fire rushing upward)

【Treatment Principles】

Clear liver and gall bladder fire, open the collaterals, and stop pain

【Treatment】

DU 20 (*bǎi huì*)	GB 20 (*fēng chí*)	PC 6 (*nèi guān*)
LI 4 (*hé gǔ*)	LV 3 (*tài chōng*)	GB 34 (*yáng líng quán*)
GB 8 (*shuài gǔ*) **(right)**	*ā shì* (local points) **(right)**	

The patient happened to come in just as the headache came on. Acupuncture was applied and it stopped his headache. On the following day, he said he only had two episodes of headache with a reduction in the level of pain. It stopped completely after three treatments. Two more acupuncture treatments were given to consolidate the effect. The follow-up found no recurrence.

【Note】

Stagnated qi of liver transforms into fire and via the exterior-interior relationship to the gall bladder transfers into that organ system. LI 4 (*hé gǔ*), LV 3 (*tài chōng*), GB 34 (*yáng líng quán*) are used to clear fire from the liver and gall bladder. GB 20 (*fēng chí*) is used to eliminate wind obstructing the channels. *Ā shì* (local points) are needled as a local treatment to stop pain. DU 20 (*bǎi huì*) clears fire by bringing it downward. PC 6 (*nèi guān*) functions to settle the heart and calm the mind. When the free flow of qi is restored to the liver, the fire will be extinguished on its own, without obstruction, there is no pain.

Sun Liu-he's Medical Records

X X, male, 37

【Chief Complaint】

A pounding pain in the forehead for several months

【Present Medical History】

Everyday the pain would start after breakfast, and gradually became worse as the morning wore on, after lunch it would get better, and as the afternoon wore on it would disappear. His stools were dry.

【Examination】

Red tongue, thin yellow coating, surging pulse

【Diagnosis】

Yangming headache (due to excess heat)

【Treatment Principles】

Reduce heat to stop pain

【Treatment】

ST 44 (*nèi tíng*)	LI 4 (*hé gǔ*)

He was cured with one week's treatment.

【Note】

The pain was in the forehead and started at *Mǎo*, which is the time when qi flows most strongly in the hand *yangming* large intestine channel. This patient's headache was due to *yangming* excess heat.

ST 44 (*nèi tíng*), is a point on the lower part of the body that is used to treat disease in the upper aspect of the body, is selected to bring down heat; as it is a *yíng*-spring point it functions to clear *yangming* heat. LI 4 (*hé gǔ*) the *yuán*-source point of the hand *yangming* large intestine channel is drained to clear heat and stop pain. This is a combination of upper and lower points that work in a synergistic fashion as each reinforces the function of the other.

If there is stabbing pain in the forehead that occurs in the evening or does not always come at regular and specific times, and is accompanied by a dark purple tongue and rough pulse, then this is a blood stasis presentation. LI 4 (*hé gǔ*) along with *shǒu miàn* (EX-HN17), as it is a local point on the forehead, which is on the affected channel, are selected for use along with BL 17 (*gé shù*), SP 10 (*xuè hǎi*), BL 40 (*wěi zhōng*). For serious cases, *nèi yíng xiāng* (EX-HN9) can be added. Of these points, LI 4 (*hé gǔ*) and *shǒu miàn* (EX-HN17) are selected according to the channel differentiation and others as used to treat the underlying pathology of blood stasis. BL 17 (*gé shù*), SP 10 (*xuè hǎi*), BL 40 (*wěi zhōng*) function to improve blood circulation to remove stasis; *nèi yíng xiāng* (EX-HN9) is an important point for treating *yangming* headaches. For stubborn headache this point is bled using a 26 or 28 gauge needle. The needle should be directed toward the base of the nose, 3~5ml of dark blood should come out.

X X, male, 26

【Chief Complaint】
Temporal headache after injury due to trauma

【Present Medical History】
This patient's headache was stabbing in nature. Half a month of acupuncture treatment in his hometown using GB 20 (*fēng chí*), SJ 5 (*wài guān*) and local points in the temporal region did not have any significant effect.

【Examination】
Blood stasis spots on the tongue, pulse was wiry and rough

【Diagnosis】
Shaoyang headache (due to blood stasis)

【Treatment Principles】
Invigorate blood, remove stasis, stop pain

【Treatment】

GB 20 (*fēng chí*)	GB 41 (*zú lín qì*)	SP 10 (*xuè hǎi*)

BL 17 (*gé shù*)

When needling GB 20 (*fēng chí*), after the patient experienced a heavy and distended feeling, the needle was rotated forward using the thumb to direct the needling sensation to the temporal region.

【Note】

This is a *shaoyang* headache, with underlying blood stasis. GB 20 (*fēng chí*) is selected to invigorate the blood and open the channels. GB 41 (*zú lín qì*), the wood point of wood channel, clears gall bladder heat to stop pain. SP 10 (*xuè hǎi*) and BL 17 (*gé shù*) are needled to remove blood stasis and stop pain.

If the headache is characterized by a sensation of being wrapped up with a bandage and accompanied with dizziness and nausea or vomiting, this is phlegm and damp stagnation type of *shaoyang* headache. This can be treated by needling from ST 8 (*tóu wéi*) through to SJ 20 (*jiǎo sūn*) with a 3 inch needle; the needling sensation should reach to the temporal region. ST 8 (*tóu wéi*) is indicated for damp and phlegm, while SJ 20 (*jiǎo sūn*) is used as a local point. RN 12 (*zhōng wǎn*) and PC 6 (*nèi guān*) are used to regulate qi, transform phlegm, eliminate dampness, and remove obstructions from the channels.

X X, female, 42

【Chief Complaint】

Hollow-like headache at the top of head for two years

【Present Medical History】

This patient's hollow-like headache at the top of head was worse with movement. Additionally, she had insomnia. While she had had many acupuncture treatments, they were not effective for her.

【Diagnosis】

Jueyin headache (due to yin deficiency of the liver and kidney)

【Treatment Principles】

Tonify the liver and kidney, remove obstructions, stop the pain

【Treatment】

| KI 1 (*yǒng quán*) | KI 3 (*tài xī*) | DU 20 (*bǎi huì*) |

The patient underwent many acupuncture treatments, which cured her problem, but it later returned. A year after stopping treatment the headaches returned. She underwent another course of treatment which brought about the same results as before.

【Note】

Vertex headache is due to liver and kidney yin deficiency. *A Handbook of Points in Verse* (*Zhǒu Hòu Gē*, 肘后歌) says: "For the headache on the top with difficulties in opening eyes, puncture KI 1 (*yǒng quán*) to stay healthy." KI 1 (*yǒng quán*) is selected here to replenish kidney water which tonifies the mother of liver, KI 3 (*tài xī*) functions to replenish the yin of liver and kidney, and DU 20 (*bǎi huì*) causes the qi to rise up to the diseased area. While only three points are used, as they directly target the yin deficiency of liver and kidney and affected channels, their effect is profound.

Summary

The head is where all the *yang* channels meet; the clear yang qi of six *fu* organs and essence of five *zang* organs all flow upward to it. Any problems with the flow of qi and blood that leads to an obstruction of the channels in the head, regardless of whether it is caused by external or internal factors will result in headache.

Headache due to external factors manifests with a quick onset and continuous pain that involves the neck and back. Wind cold headache is an example of this, it is characterized by aversion to wind and cold, with a floating and tight pulse. Headache due to wind heat includes signs of distending pain, fever and a floating and rapid pulse. Wind damp headache is characterized by a bandage-wrapped sensation in the head, accompanied by a heavy feeling of the body and limbs, fatigue, and a soggy pulse.

Headache due to internal factors manifests with slow onset and is accompanied by dizziness. Headaches due to an upsurge of liver-yang, including liver fire and liver wind, are related to kidney deficiency failing to irrigate wood or blood deficiency failing to nourish liver; these patterns manifest with a wiry pulse. Headache due to deficiency of qi and blood manifests as a dull pain with dizziness, it becomes worse when the patient is tired, the pulse is thin and weak.

For treatment, a draining method is used for excess conditions, while tonifying is adopted for deficiency conditions.

Main points: DU 20 (*băi huì*), GB 20 (*fēng chí*), *tài yáng* (EX-HN5), LI 4 (*hé gŭ*).

Frontal headache is due to involvement of the *yangming* channel; it is known as a *yangming* headache. It is treated with points such as ST 8 (*tóu wéi*), *yìn táng* (EX-HN3) and BL 2 (*cuán zhú*).

An occipital headache involves the *taiyang* channel, here it is known as a *taiyang* headache, BL 10 (*tiān zhù*), SI 3 (*hòu xī*) and BL 60 (*kūn lún*) are points that should be considered; for the intractable cases of occipital headache add BL 67 (*zhì yīn*). As is stated in *A Handbook of Points in Verse*: "Puncture BL 67 (*zhì yīn*) for the diseases of head and face."

A migraine is the headache that involves the *shaoyang* channel, thus is known as a *shaoyang* headache, GB 8 (*shuài gŭ*), SJ 5 (*wài guān*) and GB 41 (*zú lín qì*) are the points to add.

A parietal headache involves the *jueyin* channel, thus is known as a *jueyin* headache; treat it with BL 7 (*tōng tiān*) and LV 3 (*tài chōng*).

DIZZINESS (VERTIGO)

Cheng Xin-nong's Medical Records

Xia, male, 62, first visit was on May 27, 1985

【Chief Complaint】
Dizziness and nausea for 20 days

【Present Medical History】

Twenty days beforehand, the patient felt suddenly dizzy and nauseous and he had difficulty opening his eyes. He was diagnosed with cerebral arteriosclerosis, and was treated at the hospital with medication. He felt somewhat better, but he still felt dizzy in the afternoon, still had trouble opening his eyes, and his ears felt obstructed. Generally he tended to be anxious, he had a bitter taste in his mouth, dry stools, poor appetite, and thirst without desire to drink.

【Examination】

Dark red tongue, yellow and slightly thick coating, and a wiry pulse

【Diagnosis】

Dizziness (due to phlegm damp retention in middle *jiao*)

【Treatment Principles】

Calm the liver, subdue yang, transform phlegm, and regulate middle *jiao*

【Treatment】

DU 20 (*bǎi huì*)	GB 20 (*fēng chí*)	*tài yáng* (EX-HN5)
LI 4 (*hé gǔ*)	LV 3 (*tài chōng*)	GB 34 (*yáng líng quán*)
ST 36 (*zú sān lǐ*)	ST 40 (*fēng lóng*)	SP 6 (*sān yīn jiāo*)

LV 3 (*tài chōng*) and GB 34 (*yáng líng quán*) were drained. Moxibustion was applied at SP 6 (*sān yīn jiāo*). An even method was used for the remaining points.

The patient said that with the moxibustion at SP 6 (*sān yīn jiāo*) he felt warmth going from abdomen up to chest and then down to the lower abdomen. After an afternoon nap he woke up and was thirsty enough to drink five cups of water; afterwards his dizziness was greatly relieved. After 30 treatments, all his symptoms improved. He especially felt better when his abdomen and back were covered up and kept warm.

【Note】

"All wind disease and dizziness are due to disorders of the liver." This patient's problem was caused by the stagnant liver qi transforming into fire, coupled with spleen deficiency leading to dampness in the middle *jiao* obstructing the ascent of clear yang. As Zhu Dan-xi said: "Without phlegm, there will not be dizziness, in this case phlegm is brought upward by wind."

DU 20 (*bǎi huì*) is a point on the *du* vessel located in the middle of top of the head, a collateral of which enters the brain; all the vessels meet at this point, it brings up the clear yang, and disperses qi and blood. LI 4 (*hé gǔ*) and LV 3 (*tài chōng*) drain liver fire. GB 20 (*fēng chí*) helps *tài yáng* (EX-HN5) to subdue the flaring yang in the head. GB 34 (*yáng líng quán*) clears liver fire. ST 36 (*zú sān lǐ*) and SP 6 (*sān yīn jiāo*) tonify the middle *jiao* and strengthen the spleen and stomach. ST 40 (*fēng lóng*) transforms phlegm. The dizziness was cured with a month of treatment.

Wang, female, 32, first visit was on April 9, 1992

【Chief Complaint】

Feeling dizzy for more than one month

【Present Medical History】

She was diagnosed at the hospital with vestibular neuritis. She had dizziness, nausea and vomiting, a poor appetite, insomnia, neck pain, constipation, amenorrhea with scanty flow

【Examination】

Sallow complexion, pale tongue with tooth marks, white coating slightly greasy, the pulse was wiry with the proximal position being weak

【Diagnosis】

Dizziness (due to qi and blood deficiency)

【Treatment Principles】

Strengthen the spleen, harmonize the stomach, raise the clear yang, and transform turbid qi

【Treatment】

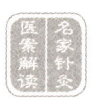

DU 14 (*dà zhuī*)	GB 20 (*fēng chí*)	BL 10 (*tiān zhù*)
tài yáng (EX-HN5)	BL 2 (*cuán zhú*)	RN 17 (*dàn zhōng*)
RN 12 (*zhōng wǎn*)	PC 6 (*nèi guān*)	BL 20 (*pí shù*)

| ST 36 (*zú sān lǐ*) | ST 40 (*fēng lóng*) | SP 6 (*sān yīn jiāo*) |

SP 4 (*gōng sūn*)

A tonifying method was applied to BL 20 (*pí shù*) and ST 36 (*zú sān lǐ*). An even method was used for the other points.

The patient's dizziness was reduced after two courses of treatment. After another two courses for consolidation, all the symptoms disappeared and she was cured.

【Note】

"Without deficiency, there will be no dizziness." The spleen and stomach are the sources that produce qi and blood. The spleen sends the clear upward. When the clear qi does not ascend, there will be dizziness. The stomach sends the turbid downward. When the turbid qi does not descend, there will be nausea, vomiting and constipation. Disharmony of the stomach causes insomnia. The amenorrhea with scanty menstrual flow is due to weakness of the middle *jiao*, thus not being able to produce sufficient qi and blood.

Summary

Xuán (眩), blurred vision, *Yùn* (晕), dizziness (vertigo). In mild cases it can be relieved by closing one's eyes, and serious cases the patient has a bodily sensation of whirling movement, the patient is unsteady on the feet, in severe cases there is vomiting. Clinically, it is commonly seen in cases of hypertension, nervous exhaustion, Meniere's disease, labyrinthitis, and hypotension. Doctors in the past say: without wind there is no dizziness, without phlegm there is no dizziness, without deficiency there is no dizziness. In practice this symptom [dizziness] is divided into these three types:

Main points: DU 20 (*bǎi huì*), GB 20 (*fēng chí*), ST 36 (*zú sān lǐ*), LV 3 (*tài chōng*).

This is a case of liver yang rising with manifestations of dizziness, tinnitus, distending pain in head, and anxiety. KI 3 (*tài xī*), LV 2 (*xíng jiān*), BL 18 (*gān shù*) and BL 23 (*shèn shù*) should be added to the treatment. LV 2 (*xíng jiān*) and BL 18 (*gān shù*) pacify liver to subdue yang. KI 3 (*tài xī*) and BL 23 (*shèn shù*) produce water to soften wood.

In the case of phlegm and dampness in the middle *jiao* with symptoms of a headache that feels like the head is wrapped with bandage, fullness in the chest, nausea and vomiting, ST 8 (*tóu wéi*), PC 6 (*nèi guān*), RN 12 (*zhōng wǎn*), ST 40 (*fēng lóng*) can also be added. ST 8 (*tóu wéi*) clears phlegm heat from the *yangming* and the other points strengthen the spleen, transform phlegm and open the chest and eliminate focal distention.

In the case of qi and blood deficiency characterized by symptoms of dizziness, blurry vision, pale complexion, and fatigue, RN 4 (*guān yuán*), ST 36 (*zú sān lǐ*) and SP 6 (*sān yīn jiāo*) should be added. ST 36 (*zú sān lǐ*) and SP 6 (*sān yīn jiāo*) replenish qi and blood; and RN 4 (*guān yuán*) strengthens the *yuán*-source qi.

FACIAL PAIN

Lu Shou-yan's Medical Record

Guo, male, 42, first visit was on October 16, 1963

【**Chief Complaint**】
Pain in the right cheek and temporal region

【**Present Medical History**】
This patient suffered from facial pain some years ago and was cured by the tapping therapy using a Seven-star needle. Recently, due to fatigue he had recurrence. The pain on the right side of face was especially worse on the lateral side of nose, warmth made it worse; the pain would start to manifest everyday in the evening. His stools were not well formed.

【**Examination**】
Swollen red tongue, white greasy coating, the pulse was soft, a bit slow and wiry.

【**Diagnosis**】
Facial pain (due to damp retained in the *yangming*)

【Treatment Principles】

Clear liver, reduce heat, transform turbidity, harmonize the collaterals

【Treatment】

tài yáng (EX-HN5)	LI 20 (*yíng xiāng*)	RN 12 (*zhōng wǎn*)
ST 6 (*jiá chē*)	SJ 17 (*yì fēng*)	LI 4 (*hé gǔ*)
ST 36 (*zú sān lǐ*)	SP 9 (*yīn líng quán*)	LV 2 (*xíng jiān*)

A tonifying method was used for ST 36 (*zú sān lǐ*) and RN 12 (*zhōng wǎn*). A draining method was used for the rest. Treatment was given once every other day. Four treatments cured him.

【Note】

The cheek is the attributed to the *yangming*. "Facial diseases are attributed to the stomach." Therefore, both flaring of fire and blockage of qi in the *yangming* channel may result in a facial pain. Clinically, it is commonly seen in elderly patients, especially those have yin deficiency with fire. Some young patients with *yangming* fire flaring due to over consumption of spicy greasy food may also suffer from facial pain. The patient here has his pain due to fatigue, his stools, pulse and tongue all show signs of spleen deficiency with dampess, only the slightly wiry pulse and red tongue indicate the presence of deficiency fire retained in the interior. It is said that deficiency fire may be stirred up by fatigue. The patient is in a profession where he has to use his head, this kind of mental work exhausted his heart blood, so heart fire stirred up liver yang, which brought dampness into the *yangming* channel. This explains why his pain always started in the late afternoon, this is when the deficient yang would float up. Professor Lu clearly differentiated the cause of this patient's condition, then treated the manifestation (*Biāo* 标) with the principle of clearing the liver to reduce heat, and treated the cause (*Běn* 本) with the strategy transforming turbidity and harmonizing the *yangming*. Hence, the patient was cured with only four treatments.

Cheng Xin-nong's Medical Record

Wang, male, 55, first visit was on September 2, 1986

【Chief Complaint】

Paroxysmal pain in the right orbital region for 2 months

【Present Medical History】

This patient's pain was like an electrical shock, it would occur once every two to three days or once a week, lasting about one minute each time. The pain would occur when he washed his face or even touched it, afterwards it was as if nothing happened.

【Examination】

Red tongue with a thin coating, wiry pulse

【Diagnosis】

Facial pain (due to liver and stomach excess fire)

【Treatment Principles】

Remove obstruction of channels, reduce fire, stop pain

【Treatment】

DU 20 (bǎi huì)	GB 14 (yáng bái)	ST 2 (sì bái)
tài yáng (EX-HN5)	SJ 23 (sī zhú kōng)	BL 2 (cuán zhú)
yú yāo (EX-HN4)	SJ 5 (wài guān)	LI 4 (hé gǔ)

Tài yáng (EX-HN5) needled through to SJ 23 (*sī zhú kōng*) and BL 2 (*cuán zhú*) needled through to *yú yāo* (EX-HN4). Other points were drained. The pain gradually stopped after five treatments.

【Note】

This patient's pain is due to liver and stomach excess fire obstructing the *shaoyang* channel. DU 20 (*bǎi huì*) awakens the spirit, opens the orifices, regulates qi and blood. LI 4 (*hé gǔ*) and SJ 5 (*wài guān*) disperse and open the qi of the *yangming* and the *shaoyang*. The others are local points used to invigorate the blood, and remove blockages from the channels to stop pain.

Summary

Facial pain is a kind of severe pain occurring in transient paroxysms with abrupt onset like an electric shock, or has an intolerable cutting or burning sensation, which lasts from several seconds to several minutes, it can occur several times a day. In modern medicine trigeminal neuralgia can have this kind of presentation. Mostly it occurs in women between the age of 40 and 60. Treatment by acupuncture involves retention of the needles. Even for secondary branch symptoms, treatment should still be aimed at the primary root cause.

Main points: GB 20 (*fēng chí*), ST 7 (*xià guān*), LI 4 (*hé gǔ*).

GB 14 (*yáng bái*) needled through to *yú yāo* (EX-HN4) and SJ 23 (*sī zhú kōng*) needled through to *yú yāo* (EX-HN4) treats orbital pain. ST 2 (*sì bái*) needled through to ST 3 (*jù liáo*) is for infraorbital pain and ST 6 (*jiá chē*) needled through to ST 4 (*dì cāng*) treats lower gum pain.

FACIAL PARALYSIS

Cheng Xin-nong's Medical Records

Hu, female, 33, first visit was on December 7, 1987

【Chief Complaint】

Facial paralysis on right side for 4 days

【Present Medical History】

Six days ago, the patient felt a distending pain on the right side of her face in the area of the mandible she treated it herself by taking *Băn Lán Gēn Chōng Jì* (Radix Isatidis Infusion). Four days ago when she got up in the morning she began to experience muscle paralysis on the right side of face, resulting in deviation of the mouth and inability to completely close the right eye. She had two acupuncture treatments in a hospital. At the time of her visit, she had headache on the right side, dream-disturbed sleep, poor and appetite; her stools and urine were normal.

【Examination】

Disappearance of wrinkles on the right side of her face, inability to completely close the eye, drooping of the mouth, inability to frown. Red tongue with a white coating and cracks in the middle of tongue, deep wiry pulse.

【Diagnosis】

Facial paralysis

【Treatment Principles】

Dispel wind, invigorate the blood, open the collaterals

【Treatment】

DU 20 (bǎi huì)	GB 20 (fēng chí)	tài yáng (EX-HN5)
RN 24 (chéng jiāng)	ST 36 (zú sān lǐ)	SP 6 (sān yīn jiāo)
LI 4 (hé gǔ)	LV 3 (tài chōng)	
Right side:	SI 18 (quán liáo)	GB 14 (yang bái)
BL 1 (jīng míng)	ST 2 (sì bái)	LI 20 (yíng xiāng)
ST 4 (dì cāng)	ST 6 (jiá chē)	

BL 1 (jīng míng) was needled with an insertion to the depth of 0.8~1.5 inches without being retained. ST 4 (dì cāng) was needled through to ST 6 (jiá chē). An even method was used for the other points.

Her problem resolved after fourteen treatments.

【Note】

Invasion of wind and blockage of channels results in the muscles being poorly nourished, thus leading to paralysis. Obstruction of qi and blood caused the mastoid pain and headache. DU 20 (bǎi huì) regulates yin and yang and circulates qi and blood. GB 20 (*fēng chí*) dispels wind and expels pathogenic factors. *Tài yáng* (EX-HN5) disperses exterior pathogenic wind. ST 36 (*zú sān lǐ*), SP 6 (*sān yīn jiāo*), LI 4 (*hé gǔ*) and LV 3 (*tài chōng*) activate the normal qi and regulate the flow of qi and blood throughout the whole body. The other points dispel wind and remove obstructions from the channels. When wind is dispelled, channels unobstructed, and muscles well nourished, paralysis will naturally on its own resolve.

Li, male, 50, first visit was on October 29, 1982

【Chief Complaint】

Deviation of mouth and eye on the right side for one day

【Present Medical History】

One day ago, the patient felt tightness on the right side of his face after exposure to wind resulting in deviation of his mouth and eye. His appetite was normal, as were urine and stools.

【Examination】

His mouth deviated to the left, his right eye was not able to close completely. Slightly red tongue with a thick, yellow coating, wiry pulse.

【Diagnosis】

Facial paralysis (due to invasion of exogenous wind)

【Treatment Principles】

Dispel wind, invigorate the blood, remove obstruction of channels

【Treatment】

DU 20 (*bǎi huì*)	GB 20 (*fēng chí*)	LI 4 (*hé gǔ*)
Right side:	GB 14 (*yáng bái*)	ST 2 (*sì bái*)
SI 18 (*quán liáo*)	ST 4 (*dì cāng*)	ST 6 (*jiá chē*)

ST 4 (*dì cāng*) was needled through to ST 6 (*jiá chē*). An even method was applied to the other points. With two weeks' treatment, he was basically cured.

【Note】

The facial region is mostly nourished by the *yangming* and *shaoyang* channels. Pathogenic wind invades when there is a deficiency of channels, thus blocking the qi causing a lack of nourishment to the muscles, resulting in paralysis. The treatment principles to follow are to invigorate the blood, dispel wind, and remove obstruction from the channels. The points of the *yangming* and *shaoyang* channels are selected.

Yang Jie-bin's Medical Records

Luo, male, 16, first visit was on March 5, 1995

【Chief Complaint】

Deviation of the mouth and eye to the left side for 2 months

【Present Medical History】

Two months ago the patient's mouth and eye began to deviate to the left, there was accompanying numbness of the facial region, and hypogeusesthesia. He received treatment of Chinese and western medicine and acupuncture, but there was no improvement.

【Examination】

Deviation of the right eye and drooping of angle of mouth, numbness and twitching of facial muscles, disappearance of wrinkles, inability to frown and fill the cheek with air, palpebral fissure 1.5 cm, nasolabial groove becoming shallow, philtrum deviating to the left side, tenderness in the mastoid region, dark red tongue, with a thin white coating, thin, wiry pulse.

【Diagnosis】

Facial paralysis

【Treatment Principles】

Remove obstructions from the channels, strengthen the upright to dispel pathogens

【Treatment】

Main points:	palpebral conjunctiva of right eye		buccal mucosa of right side
Group 1:	ST 4 (dì cāng)	ST 6 (jiá chē)	GB 14 (yáng bái)
	qiú hòu (EX-HN7)	LI 20 (yíng xiāng)	DU 26 (rén zhōng)
	LI 4 (hé gǔ)		
Group 2:	LI 19 (kǒu hé liáo)	SI 18 (quán liáo)	yì zhōng (EX-HN18)
	ST 1 (chéng qì)	ST 36 (zú sān lǐ)	LU 7 (liè quē)

Group 1: ST 4 (dì cāng) needled through to ST 6 (jiá chē). Group 2: LI 19 (kǒu hé liáo) needled through to SI 18 (quán liáo). The palpebral conjunctiva of the right eye and buccal mucosa of the right side were pricked and bled. An even method was applied to the other points. Cupping for 5 to 10 minutes at ST 7 (xià guān) after needling. Treatment was given once everyday or every other day. The symptoms were significantly reduced after one course of treatment. The patient was basically cured with 15 treatments.

【Note】

This case of facial paralysis was caused by a weakness of the defensive qi, and a disharmony between the ying-nutritive wei-defensive qi, allowing wind cold invasion to obstruct the channels leading to muscular malnutrition; thus paralysis. Plain Questions - On Adjusting the Channels by Needling (Sù Wèn: Tiáo Jīng Lùn, 素问·调经论) says: "For disease in blood, treat the collaterals." Pricking to cause bleeding is aimed at removing obstructions of qi and blood and dispelling wind. Professor Yang utilizes bleeding and cupping after needling. Warming and nourishing the muscles, unobstructing the channels and regulating qi and blood cures the paralysis.

> **Bleeding the palpebral conjunctiva and buccal mucosa** (affected side):
> To bleed the palpebral conjunctiva:
> Expose the palpebral conjunctiva, disinfect with sterilized cotton ball dipped, prick the tarsus 5~7 times with a #28 filiform needle or a thin three-edged needle or until there is a little bleeding.

> *To bleed the buccal mucosa:*
> *The patient is asked to open their mouth to expose the buccal mucosa. Disinfect with alcohol cotton ball. Prick the buccal mucosa several times with a 15 cm three-edged needle once every 0.5 cm in distance, till there is a little bleeding.*

Song, male, 34

【Chief Complaint】
Deviation of mouth and eye on the left side

【Present Medical History】
Two years ago, the patient had facial paralysis on the left side due to invasion of wind cold. Acupuncture, physical therapy, and medication, relieved his symptoms, but did not completely cure him. Recently the condition worsened due to fatigue and being caught in rain.

【Examination】
Disappearance of wrinkles on the left side, left mimetic paralysis, inability to frown, blow out the cheek, and show the teeth or whistle, incomplete closure of eyelids, left nasolabial groove becoming shallow, philtrum deviating to the right side, dribbling of water when drinking, and pain in the mastoid region. Pale red tongue with a thin white coating, deep and thready pulse.

【Diagnosis】
Facial paralysis

【Treatment Principles】
Remove obstructions, activate blood, regulate *ying* - nutrient *wei* - defense

【Treatment】

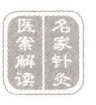

Left Side:	palpebral conjunctiva and buccal mucosa		
	ST 4 (*dì cāng*)	ST 6 (*jiá chē*)	GB 14 (*yáng bái*)
	yú yāo (EX-HN4)	LI 20 (*yíng xiāng*)	ST 2 (*sì bái*)

Both sides: LI 4 (*hé gǔ*)   ST 36 (*zú sān lǐ*)

The palpebral conjunctiva of left eye and buccal mucosa of left side were bled. Each treatment involved two to four facial points being punctured and needled through to other points. ST 4 (*dì cāng*) to ST 6 (*jiá chē*), GB 14 (*yáng bái*) to *yú yāo* (EX-HN4), and ST 2 (*sì bái*) to LI 20 (*yíng xiāng*). Moxibustion was applied for five minutes after needling. Perpendicular insertions at LI 4 (*hé gǔ*) and ST 36 (*zú sān lǐ*) with an even method were applied.

Treatment was given once every day, with 10 treatments constituting one course. His condition improved after one month, and he was clinically cured after half a year of continuous treatment.

【Note】

This patient's facial paralysis was due to fatigue, complicated by invasion of wind cold blocking the facial region, with stagnation of qi and blood causing malnutrition of muscles. Bleeding the conjunctiva and buccal mucosa activated the blood circulation, and removed obstructions from channels. Moxibustion after needling ST 4 (*dì cāng*), ST 6 (*jiá chē*), GB 14 (*yáng bái*), *yú yāo* (EX-HN4), LI 20 (*yíng xiāng*), LI 4 (*hé gǔ*), and ST 36 (*zú sān lǐ*) regulated the qi and blood, harmonized the *ying* - nutritive and *wei* - defensive thus nourishing the muscles. For stubborn cases of facial paralysis, self massage and functional exercises can help to improve the recovery.

Summary

Facial paralysis, is exemplified by deviation of the mouth and eye; lack of motor impairment of the extremities or loss of consciousness, it is mostly caused by an invasion of wind in the facial region, or phlegm retention in the channels, causing malnutrition of the facial muscles, or secondary to tympanitis or herpes. Points of the *yangming* channels of the hand and foot are primarily selected and needled with an even method.

Commonly used points: GB 20 (*fēng chí*), SJ 17 (*yì fēng*), ST 2 (*sì bái*), SI 18 (*quán liáo*), ST 4 (*dì cāng*), ST 6 (*jiá chē*), SJ 5 (*wài guān*), and LI 4 (*hé gǔ*).

Add *tài yáng* (EX-HN5) for headache; add GB 14 (*yáng bái*) and BL 2 (*cuán zhú*) for inability to frown; puncture BL 1 (*jīng míng*) as deep as 0.8~1.5 inch without retaining for incomplete closure of eyelid; add LI 20 (*yíng xiāng*) for inability to wrinkle the nose; include DU 26 (*rén zhōng*) for philtrum deviation; add ST 3 (*jù liáo*) for inability to show the teeth; add LV 3 (*tài chōng*) for twitching of the mouth and eyes; add GB 12 (*wán gǔ*) for mastoid pain; needle ST 40 (*fēng lóng*) for profuse phlegm.

WIND STROKE

Lu Shou-yan's Medical Record

Chen, male, 45, first visit was on May 29, 1963

【Chief Complaint】

Numbness of the left arm

【Present Medical History】

In the past he suffered a stroke. Three months ago, he again had a stroke. While his symptoms were improving and his blood pressure tended toward normal, the left shoulder, elbow, wrist, and fingers were numb, contracted, and with motor impairment. He had accompanying dizziness, migraine on the right side, palpitations, nausea, a preference for warmth and a dislike of cold.

【Examination】

The right distal and middle pulse were wiry and slippery, the Chi pulse was big; the left pulse was soggy, thin and wiry. Pulse of GB 4 (*hán yàn*) region: right stronger than left. Pulse of ST 42 (*chōng yáng*) region: strong. Pulse of LV 3 (*tài chōng*) region: wiry thready. Pulse of KI 3 (*tài xī*) region: even. His tongue had a thin slippery coating.

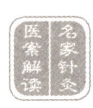

【Diagnosis】

Wind stroke with channels and collaterals being attacked (due to water deficiency and wood excess)

【Treatment Principles】

Replenish water to soften liver

【Treatment】

①	GB 4 (*hán yàn*)	GB 20 (*fēng chí*)	LV 3 (*tài chōng*)
	ST 40 (*fēng lóng*)	KI 3 (*tài xī*)	KI 7 (*fù liū*)

KI 3 (*tài xī*) and KI 7 (*fù liū*) were treated with tonifying method. Other points treated with an even method.

②	LI 15 (*jiān yú*)	LI 14 (*bì nào*)	LI 10 (*shǒu sān lǐ*)
	LI 4 (*hé gǔ*)	SJ 5 (*wài guān*)	*bā xié* (EX-UE9)

Bā xié (EX-UE9) on the right side was drained; on the left side tonified. Manipulation: mainly rotating, secondarily lifting-thrusting.

Twelve treatments constituted one course. The patient was given one course of treatment, and then allowed to rest for two weeks. After which the second course was given, followed by another two weeks of rest. Finally, the third course of treatment was performed. When the left and right pulses were balanced, only points from the second group were used on the left side, using a draining method to dispel pathogenic factors, and to strengthen the resistance. Herbal medicine applied externally was used in combination with the acupuncture.

【Note】

This patient was nearly 50 years old. His kidney qi was declining, resulting in the water being deficient and the wood being excess. He was overweight, and constitutionally qi deficient, phlegmy and damp. Because of work that requires hard mental work, the internal fire flared up, bringing phlegm damp upward, thus obstructing the channels and collaterals. The pulse was stronger and bigger on the right side pointing to there being excess on the right and deficiency on the left. Professor Lu drained the right side and tonified the left to balance yin and yang.

Point group ① aims to treat the root cause of his disease. GB 4 (*hán yàn*) and GB 20 (*fēng chí*) are drained to stop the upward flow of deficient yang; thus clearing turbidity from the head. Draining LV 3 (*tài chōng*) pacified liver, subduing yang. Draining ST 40 (*fēng lóng*) transforms phlegm. Tonifying KI 3 (*tài xī*) and KI 7 (*fù liū*) replenishes water which moistens wood.

Point group ②, was selected mostly from the affected channels, the aim is to remove obstructions from the channels and collaterals, and balance yin and yang. Because the right pulse is bigger than that of the left, the right side was drained and the left was tonified.

Yang Jia-san's Medical Record

Zhu, male, 58, first visit was on August 4, 1986

【Chief Complaint】
The right side weakness for 6 days

【Present Medical History】
Six days ago, due to emotional factors the patient began to have stiffness of tongue, right arm numbness, and right side body weakness. Use of herbal medicine controlled his condition and arrested further pathological development. Now he had a distended feeling in his head, dizziness, weakness on the right side of his body, especially the right arm, along with slurred speech, tongue stiffness, distention and dryness of the eyes, a dry mouth without desire to drink, and difficulties in falling asleep.

【Examination】

Blood pressure fluctuated between 130-150/80-110 mmHg. Dark red tongue with a white moist coating, wiry slightly slippery pulse.

【Diagnosis】

Wind stroke (attack on channels and collaterals) (due to liver yang transforming into wind)

【Treatment Principles】

Replenish yin, subdue yang, calm the mind

【Treatment】

DU 21 (*qián dǐng*)	DU 19 (*hòu dǐng*)	DU 20 (*bǎi huì*)
BL 7 (*tōng tiān*)	GB 20 (*fēng chí*)	LI 4 (*hé gǔ*)
LU 7 (*liè quē*)	SJ 6 (*zhī gōu*)	GB 39 (*jué gǔ*)
LV 3 (*tài chōng*)		

DU 21 (*qián dǐng*), DU 19 (*hòu dǐng*), DU 20 (*bǎi huì*), BL 7 (*tōng tiān*) were tonified with mild stimulation. LU 7 (*liè quē*), SJ 6 (*zhī gōu*), GB 39 (*jué gǔ*), LV 3 (*tài chōng*) were tonified with medium stimulation; the other points were drained with medium stimulation.

After three months of treatment the numbness on his right side disappeared and his speech was basically normal.

【Note】

This is a syndrome of yin deficiency and yang hyperactivity transforming into wind; there is upper excess and lower deficiency. The treatment principle is to replenish yin, subdue yang, and extinguish wind, clearing the upper, tonify the lower and calm the mind.

The head points DU 21 (*qián dǐng*), DU 19 (*hòu dǐng*), DU 20 (*bǎi huì*), and BL 7 (*tōng tiān*) are used to replenish marrow, strengthen brain and calm the mind. GB 20 (*fēng chí*) is needled to dispel wind of the upper *jiao*. LI 4 (*hé gǔ*) and ST 36 (*zú sān lǐ*) to remove obstruction from the intestines to aid in the clean ascending and the turbid descending. LI 11 (*qū chí*) and ST 36 (*zú sān lǐ*) are used to bring down counterflow qi. LI 4 (*hé gǔ*) and LV 3 (*tài chōng*) are *yuán*-source points, they function to soften liver, stop wind, and replenish yin to clear heat. LU 7 (*liè quē*) induces kidney water to nourish genuine yin, combined with GB 39 (*jué gǔ*) they increase kidney essence. GB 39 (*jué gǔ*) and LV 3 (*tài chōng*) function to increase liver and kidney essence. Thus, the lower is tonified and the upper is cleared.

Cheng Xin-nong's Medical Record

Wang, female, 73, first visit was on October 31, 1986

【Chief Complaint】
Weakness of the right limbs for two days

【Present Medical History】
Two days ago, the patient got angry with her family and suddenly had weakness of her right limbs and sluggish movement. She presented with weakness of the right limbs, sluggish movement, irritability, dry mouth, poor appetite, her sleep was fine, she had no dizziness or tinnitus, but she did have shortness of breath on exertion, and sometimes incontinence of urine.

【Examination】
Tongue tip red, dry yellow coating, deep thready pulse, proximal position especially weak

【Diagnosis】
Signs of wind stroke (due to liver and kidney deficiency)

【Treatment Principles】
Tonify the liver and kidney, harmonize qi and blood

【Treatment】

DU 20 (*bǎi huì*)	GB 20 (*fēng chí*)	RN 4 (*guān yuán*)
LI 4 (*hé gǔ*)	LV 3 (*tài chōng*)	ST 36 (*zú sān lǐ*)
SP 6 (*sān yīn jiāo*)	KI 3 (*tài xī*)	KI 1 (*yǒng quán*)
Right side:	LI 15 (*jiān yú*)	LI 11 (*qū chí*)

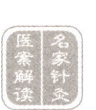

SJ 5 (*wài guān*)	GB 34 (*yáng líng quán*)	GB 39 (*xuán zhōng*)

GB 20 (*fēng chí*) and LV 3 (*tài chōng*) were drained. RN 4 (*guān yuán*), ST 36 (*zú sān lǐ*), SP 6 (*sān yīn jiāo*), and KI 3 (*tài xī*) were tonified; an even method was used for the others.

After three treatments, there was a reduction of numbness and weakness of the right limbs and movement was free from sluggishness. Her condition stabilized with 10 treatments. The follow-up found no recurrence. On July 6, 1987, she felt weakness in her lower limbs. This was diagnosed as kidney deficiency, eight treatments cured her.

【Note】

This patient is elderly with liver and kidney deficiency, qi and blood insufficiency, and anger issues that stagnated her liver qi, which caused lack of nourishment to the limbs. Because of the kidney yin deficiency, body fluids fail to distribute upward, so there is dryness of the mouth. Yin deficiency leads to internal heat, so there are signs of a red tongue with yellow coating, and a thready, rapid pulse. Kidney deficiency leads to an inability to hold the qi, so there is shortness of breath on exertion. The urinary bladder is disharmonious owing to the kidney qi not being firmed, so there is incontinence. This is a syndrome of liver and kidney deficiency.

DU 20 (*bǎi huì*) is used to regulate yin and yang, and circulate qi and blood. GB 20 (*fēng chí*) dispels wind. LV 3 (*tài chōng*) pacifies liver and subdues yang. RN 4 (*guān yuán*) functions to tonify *yuán*-source qi. ST 36 (*zú sān lǐ*) strengthens the middle *jiao*. SP 6 (*sān yīn jiāo*) replenishes yin to subdue yang. KI 3 (*tài xī*) functions to replenish water which irrigates wood. KI 1 (*yǒng quán*) is needled to conduct fire downward. LI 15 (*jiān yú*), LI 11 (*qū chí*), SJ 5 (*wài guān*), LI 4 (*hé gǔ*), GB 34 (*yáng líng quán*), and GB 39 (*xuán zhōng*) all remove obstructions from the channels and balance yin and yang.

Shi Xue-min's Medical Record

Li, male, 56, first visit was on April 10, 1992

【Chief Complaint】

Hemiplegia of the right side for 4 days

【Present Medical History】

The patient had hemiplegia of the right side for four days, he could not walk without help, and the right hand was too weak to grasp anything.

【Examination】

Clear consciousness, slurred speech, dull expression; second and third degree myodynamia of limbs on the right side, CT of the head showed "cerebral infarction in the left basal region," the tongue was pale with a white coating, wiry pulse.

【Diagnosis】

Wind stroke (due to attack on channels and collaterals)

【Treatment Principles】

Wake the brain and open the orifices, nourish the liver and kidney, dredge the channels and collaterals

【Treatment】

| PC 6 (nèi guān) | DU 26 (rén zhōng) | SP 6 (sān yīn jiāo) |
| HT 1 (jí quán) | LU 5 (chǐ zé) | BL 40 (wěi zhōng) |

The technique of restoring consciousness and opening the orifices was adopted. First PC 6 (nèi guān) was bilaterally needled perpendicularly 1~1.5 inches using a lifting-thrusting and rotating movement for one minute, then DU 26 (rén zhōng) was needled, five minutes after insertion, a lifting-thrusting like sparrow picking motion was employed till the patient was tearing. SP 6 (sān yīn jiāo) was inserted 1~1.5 inches at the posterior border of the tibia with a 45° angle lifting-thrusting movement that caused the lower limb to contract three 3 times. HT 1 (jí quán) inserted 1~1.5 inches perpendicularly and with a lifting-thrusting motion which caused the upper limb to contract three times. LU 5 (chǐ zé) was needled in the same way as HT 1 (jí quán). With the patient in a supine position and leg stretched out

BL 40 (*wěi zhōng*) was needled using a one inch needle employing a lifting-thrusting motion which caused the lower limb to contract three times.

After the first treatment, the patient could come for treatment by himself with the help of walking stick; he said his right limbs were much stronger. One week of treatment succeeded in him being able to walk normally.

【Note】

In the treatment of windstroke, it is necessary to dispel wind and remove obstructions from the channels and collaterals; points from the *yangming* channels, which are full of qi and blood, are often selected for this purpose. Professor Shi has put forward that closing of the orifices and hiding of the spirit was the root pathology based on the location of the disease based on the concepts of modern medicine. He holds that when the orifices are closed the spirit has no place to abide, so limbs were soft and speech slurred. Waking the brain and opening the orifices should be the principle for treatment. Using the theory of liver and kidney yin deficiency as conceived of by doctors of previous generations, he treated windstroke with waking the brain and opening the orifices as the main principle along with unobstructing the channels of brain and replenishing liver and kidney yin.

Main points: PC 6 (*nèi guān*), DU 26 (*rén zhōng*), SP 6 (*sān yīn jiāo*).

Supplementary points: HT 1 (*jí quán*), LU 5 (*chǐ zé*), BL 40 (*wěi zhōng*).

PC 6 (*nèi guān*), the *luò*-connecting point and confluent point of the *yinwei mai*, nourishes the heart, calms the mind, circulates qi and blood. DU 26 (*rén zhōng*), an intersecting point of the *du* vessel with the *yangming* channels, restores consciousness and induces resuscitation. SP 6 (*sān yīn jiāo*), the intersecting point of the three yin channels of the foot replenishes kidney essence to fill up marrow; when the brain marrow is ample, the mind has an abode within which to dwell. HT 1 (*jí quán*), LU 5 (*chǐ zé*), and BL 40 (*wěi zhōng*) are located on joints where the channel qi converges; they have a strong effect in circulating channel qi to improve movement of the limbs.

Added points: GB 20 (*fēng chí*), SJ 17 (*yì fēng*), and GB 12 (*wán gǔ*) for dysphagia; *jīn jīn* (EX-HN12), *yù yè* (EX-HN13) for aphasia; LI 4 (*hé gǔ*) for inability to move fingers; others used accordingly for symptomatic relief.

Manipulation of added points: GB 20 (*fēng chí*), SJ 17 (*yì fēng*), and GB

12 (*wán gǔ*) were punctured towards the Adam's apple with a 2~2.5 inch insertion, and tonified by rotating the needle with small amplitude and high frequency for half a minute. LI 4 (*hé gǔ*) was needled towards LI 3 (*sān jiān*) to the lower border of the 2nd metacarpal bone using a lifting-thrusting motion to drain causing the index finger to contract. *Jīn jīn* (EX-HN12), *yù yè* (EX-HN13) was bled.

Professor Shi stressed that for good therapeutic results the technique for each point should be strictly followed. Many patients with channel and collateral obstruction due to this kind of attack got immediate results, with a decrease in the duration of the disease.

Bo Zhi-yun's Medical Record

Sun, male, 65

【Chief Complaint】

Motor impairment of the right limbs and slurring of speech for eight months, worse in the past two days

【Present Medical History】

Lacking any obvious reasons the patient began to have motor impairment of the right limbs, especially the arm; along with slurring of speech and salivation, he did not have a headache, but did experience nausea and vomiting. A CT of the head showed cerebral infarction of the left temporal lobe. With treatment his symptoms improved, but the motor impairment of the right limbs still existed; the arm could only be partially lifted, and he required the aid of a stick to walk. Two days beforehand, he was hospitalized again as his motor impairment became worse and he could not speak.

【Examination】

Motor impairment of the right limbs, edema of the distal right arm; head CT showing "a large shadow in the left temporal lobe, latent image of low density in the right corona radiata region," giving the impression of "remote infarction focused in the left temporal lobe, and ischemic changes

of the right corona radiata region." He had a pale tongue with a white greasy coating, and a deep slippery pulse.

【Diagnosis】

Wind stroke (attack on channels and collaterals) (due to spleen and kidney yang deficiency)

【Treatment Principles】

Tonify spleen and kidney, transform dampness and phlegm

【Treatment】

Abdominal acupuncture: *Conduct* **qi** *to its primary source*:

RN 12 (*zhōng wǎn*)	RN 10 (*xià wǎn*)	RN 6 (*qì hǎi*)	RN 4 (*guān yuán*)
Abdominal 4 gates:	Bilateral:	ST 24 (*huá ròu mén*)	ST 26 (*wài líng*)
Upper rheumatism point	Upper rheumatism lateral point		RN 8 (*shén què*)

Conduct **qi** *to its primary source*: insert needle to the earth level. Abdominal four gates: insert needle to the human level. Rheumatism points: insert needle to the heaven level with triangular needling added. Moxibustion was done at RN 8 (*shén què*) for 40 minutes.

Treatment was given once a day, five times a week, 10 treatments constituted one course. After 10 treatments, the hand swelling was greatly reduced, another 10 treatments and it completely disappeared; no recurrence in two months.

【Note】

This patient was treated with the abdominal acupuncture invented by Professor Bo Zhi-yun. This theory takes the point RN 8 (*shén què*) as the key to regulating the system. RN 8 (*shén què*) formed in the embryo stage, is the earliest regulating system of the human body and the mother of the channel system, it distributes qi and blood to the whole body and regulates the macroscopic aspect of the human body. Owing to the characteristics of abdominal anatomical structure, RN 8 (*shén què*) bifurcates into two in the process of gestational formation. One aspect is located shallowly in the abdominal wall, it regulates the whole body; this is known as peripheral system. The other is located deeply in the abdominal wall, it regulates the viscera; it is known as the visceral system. In abdominal acupuncture, the system of channels is a holo-image in the shape of turtle, with RN 8 (*shén què*) as its center, RN 12 (*zhōng wǎn*) as the top, RN 4 (*guān yuán*) as the tail, and SP 15 (*dà héng*) making up the lateral sides. On the arm, the **upper rheumatism point** is located 0.5 inch superolateral to ST 24 (*huá ròu mén*), and the **upper rheumatism lateral point** is 1.0 inch lateral to ST 24 (*huá ròu mén*). On lower limb, the **lower rheumatism point** is located 0.5 inch infralateral to ST 26 (*wài líng*), and the **lower rheumatism lower point** is 1.0 inch lateral to ST 27 (*dà jù*). KI 17 (*shāng qū*) is seen as the turtle's neck, KI 14 (*sì mǎn*) as starting from sacrococcyx. The abdominal *Eight-region* (*Bā Kuò*, 八廓) system, uses the image of the *post heaven Eight-diagram* (*Hòu Tiān Bā Guà*, 后天八卦) to regulate the viscera. On it, RN 12 (*zhōng wǎn*) is fire (*lí* 离) it controls the heart and small intestine; RN 4 (*guān yuán*) is water (*kǎn* 坎) it controls kidney and urine bladder; the left **upper rheumatism point** is earth (*kūn* 坤) controls the spleen and stomach; the left SP 15 (*dà héng*) is lake (*duì* 兑) dominating the lower *jiao*; the left **lower rheumatism point** is heaven (*qián* 乾) it controls the lung and large intestine; the right **upper rheumatism point** is wind (*xùn* 巽) it controls the liver and middle *jiao*; the right SP 15 (*dà héng*) is thunder (*zhèn* 震) it controls the liver and gall bladder; the right **lower rheumatism point** is mountain (*gèn* 艮) it controls the upper *jiao*. The points in each region have special therapeutic functions for their corresponding *zang-fu* organs and play an important role in the balancing of the internal organs.

In the theory of the traditional system of channels, RN 12 (*zhōng wǎn*) is the Front-*mù* of the stomach and influential point of the *fu* organs. RN 10 (*xià wǎn*) is the intersecting point of the *ren* vessel with the foot *taiyin* spleen channel. RN 4 (*guān yuán*) is Front-*mù* of the small intestine and intersects with the *ren* vessel and the three foot yin channels, like RN 6 (*qì hǎi*) it is a tonification point. ST 24 (*huá ròu mén*) and ST 26 (*wài líng*) are points of the foot *yangming* channel. Therefore, needling RN 12 (*zhōng wǎn*), RN 10 (*xià wǎn*), RN 6 (*qì hǎi*), RN 4 (*guān yuán*) and the abdominal four gates (ST 24 and ST 26) functions to conduct qi to its primary source, replenish yang qi of the spleen and kidney, regulate qi of the spleen and stomach, and strengthen the spleen to transform phlegm. When yang qi is strong, water and dampness are removed; when the spleen is strong phlegm cannot be formed. In the recovery stage of cerebral vascular accident, qi and blood have been consumed and are deficient. The spleen and kidney are weak; mostly this is a deficiency of qi. This patient in this study has edema in the distal right arm, this points to a condition of qi deficiency, which fails to circulate water so there is phlegm retention in the collaterals. Abdominal acupuncture is more effective in regulating qi and blood to remove obstructions from the channels in the affected areas. Moxibustion is a good supplement to promote qi and blood circulation. So the therapeutic effect is beneficial.

> **Conduct qi to its primary source**: it is composed of RN 12 (zhōng wǎn), RN 10 (xià wǎn), RN 6 (qì hǎi) and RN 4 (guān yuán). Of them, RN 12 (zhōng wǎn) and RN 10 (xià wǎn) act on middle jiao, regulating ascending and descending of qi. Because the lung channel of hand taiyin originates from the middle jiao at RN 12 (zhōng wǎn), needling it helps the lung in its ability to descend qi. RN 6 (qì hǎi) is the sea of qi, RN 4 (guān yuán) tonifies the kidney to consolidate the root. The kidney stores the primorial yúan - source qi, and relies on nourishment from post-natal qi. Use of these points is said to conduct qi to its primary source. The Classic of Difficulties - The Fourth Difficulty (Nàn Jīng: Sì Nàn, 难经·四难) says: "Heart and lung exhale, kidney and liver inhale." These four points function well to treat heart and lung, regulate spleen and stomach, and tonify liver and kidney.
>
> **Abdominal four gates**: it is composed of bilateral ST 24 (huá ròu mén) and ST 26 (wài líng). ST 24 (huá ròu mén) treats the upper portion of the body and upper limbs, while ST 26 (wài líng) treats lower the abdomen and lower limbs. Together they function to regulate qi and blood, circulate channel qi to the extremities, and distribute zang-fu qi to the whole body; they are indicated in whole body diseases. Used together with **Conducting qi to kidney (primary source)** or **Abdominal heaven-earth acupuncture**, it is very effective in unobstructing the fu organs.
>
> **Rheumatism points**: Professor Bo's experiential points. The **upper rheumatism point** is 0.5 inch superolateral to ST 24 (huá ròu mén). The **upper rheumatism lateral point** is 1.0 inch lateral to ST 24 (huá ròu mén). The **lower rheumatism point** is 0.5 inch infralateral to ST 26 (wài líng). The **lower rheumatism lower point** is 1.0 inch lateral to ST 27 (dà jù). They reduce swelling to stop pain, used in conjunction with SP 15 (dà héng) they function to dispel wind, lubricate the joints, and remove blood stasis. For treatment of the shoulder and elbow, the upper rheumatism point may be used singly, as can the lower rheumatism points for treatment of the lower extremities.

Yang Jie-bin's Medical Record

Li, female, 55

【Chief Complaint】

Her family reports that she suddenly fell down and lost consciousness for half a day

【Present Medical History】

The patient suffered from blurred vision and dizziness for many years and sometimes experienced numbness in her fingers. She was diagnosed with hypertension. She was overworked on the day and had a stroke. She fell down and lost consciousness, there was a phlegm gurgling sound in her throat, her left limbs seized up, her eyes were open and staring and her month was closed.

【Examination】

Unconsciousness, staring eyes, closed mouth, flushed face, phlegm gurgling in throat, abrupt respiration, BP 160/130 mm Hg, pale red tongue with a yellow sticky coating, slippery and rapid pulse.

【Diagnosis】

Wind stroke (due to attack on *zang-fu* organs, tense syndrome)

【Treatment Principles】

Promote resuscitation, pacify liver to stop wind, resolve phlegm, clear fire

【Treatment】

Five centers	DU 26 (*rén zhōng*)	*jǐng*-well points
ST 40 (*fēng lóng*)	LI 4 (*hé gǔ*)	LV 3 (*tài chōng*)

"Five centers" and *jǐng*-well points were bled; DU 26 (*rén zhōng*) was needled with a thick filiform needle and manipulated with sparrow picking method for 10 minutes; ST 40 (*fēng lóng*), LI 4 (*hé gǔ*) and LV 3 (*tài chōng*) strongly drained.

The needles were retained for 30 minutes and manipulated once every five minutes. After the first treatment her breathing normalized and restlessness resolved. On the following day, the same treatment was applied and she regained consciousness. With another three treatments given in succession, her left limbs regained some ability to move. Acupuncture was continued for three months after which she regained normal movement of her limbs.

【Note】

This is a case of liver yang transforming into fire and producing wind, wind brought phlegm damp upward disturbing the brain and flowing to the channels and collaterals; thus wind stroke, tense syndrome. First-aid treatment should be given as quickly as possible. Concerning differentiation, there are two types: flaccid and tense. These syndromes must be clearly differentiated. In this case the patient's eyes are staring, the mouth is agape with clenched jaws, stiff limbs, coarse breathing, flushed face, and a big floating pulse; this is qi and fire flaring upward. When phlegm is rattling in the throat, it is an excess tense syndrome. Promoting resuscitation and clearing heat are the primary treatment principles. Bleeding the "five centers" is a strong resuscitative treatment for patients who are unconscious. DU 26 (*rén zhōng*), LI 4 (*hé gǔ*) and *shí xuān* (EX-UE11) are used to restore consciousness. ST 40 (*fēng lóng*) sends qi down and transforms phlegm. LV 3 (*tài chōng*) is used to pacify the liver and extinguish wind.

Five centers, as used by Professor Yang Jie-bin, are composed of DU 20 (*bǎi huì*), PC 8 (*láo gōng*) and KI 1 (*yǒng quán*). These "centers" one in the brain, two in the palms and two in the soles are useful in restoring consciousness and excellent in clearing heat.

Summary

Wind stroke is a commonly seen disease in the acupuncture clinic. In modern medicine it refers to a cerebrovascular accident. Its root cause is a decline of the normal qi. This disease, while it centers in the brain, also involves the heart, liver, spleen, and kidney. The pathogenesis is due to a deficiency of the normal qi, coupled with disorders of qi and blood, retention of wind, fire, phlegm, and stasis in channels and collaterals.

When beginning to treat the immediate aftermath of wind stroke, eight points from yang channels are always selected: LI 15 (*jiān yú*), LI 11 (*qū chí*), SJ 5 (*wài guān*), LI 4 (*hé gǔ*), GB 30 (*huán tiào*), GB 34 (*yáng líng quán*), GB 39 (*xuán zhōng*), LV 3 (*tài chōng*). Generally, an even method is adopted. Yang dominates movement, so points of the yang channels are good to restore movement to the limbs.

In the later stage, points of the yin channels are selected as well. Points such as LU 5 (*chǐ zé*), PC 6 (*nèi guān*), SP 6 (*sān yīn jiāo*), KI 3 (*tài xī*) are used to circulate qi and blood, and to balance yin and yang. Most patients recover to some degree with a few courses of treatment.

For numbness (*Má Mù* 麻木) of the limbs, to regulate channels and remove obstructions for the upper limbs needle SJ 5 (*wài guān*) and SI 3 (*hòu xī*), and use GB 32 (*zhōng dú*) and GB 39 (*xuán zhōng*) for the lower limbs. ST 36 (*zú sān lǐ*) and SP 6 (*sān yīn jiāo*) are selected to replenish qi and blood as qi deficiency is the cause of (*Má* 麻) and blood deficiency the cause of (*Mù* 木). Tonifying method should be used. This illness requires a long course of treatment.

LOW BACK PAIN

Yang Yong-xuan's Medical Record

Mei, male, 46

【Chief Complaint】
Low back pain due to sprain for one week

【Present Medical History】

This patient had back pain for many years. Recently it was made worse due to lumbar sprain, which was exasperated by coughing or turning the body. Treatment by oral adminstration of herbs and use of topical herbs were without effect.

【Examination】

Patient looked tired. His tongue coating was thin and greasy, and the pulse was thin and slippery.

【Diagnosis】

Acute lumbar sprain (due to injury of the *du* vessel, the sea of yang channels)

【Treatment Principles】

Remove obstructions from the channels, dispel blood stasis

【Treatment】

DU 26 (*shuǐ gōu*)	BL 40 (*wěi zhōng*)	BL 24 (*qì hǎi shù*)

Draining method by use of rotating needle. After needling, cupping was applied to BL 24 (*qì hǎi shù*). The patient was treated once every other day. Four treatments cured the problem.

【Note】

Acute lumbar sprain is commonly seen in the acupuncture department. This patient injured his *du* vessel. Qi stagnation and blood stasis are the cause of the pain. *Jade Dragon Verse* (*Yù Lóng Gē*, 玉龙歌) says that DU 26 (*shuǐ gōu*) should be drained for spinal pain and BL 40 (*wěi zhōng*) can be used to treat diseases of the lumbar region. Here, DU 26 (*shuǐ gōu*) is used to regulate counterflow qi of the *du* vessel. BL 40 (*wěi zhōng*) regulates the qi of the foot *taiyang* bladder channel. Needling and cupping BL 24 (*qì hǎi shù*) warms and regulates both qi and blood in the low back. The pain is stopped when obstruction is removed.

Record in *Acupuncture - Moxibustion for Difficult Diseases* (*Qí Nán Zá Bìng Zhēn Jiǔ Zhì Liáo*)

He, female, 50, first visit was on January 18, 1999

【Chief Complaint】

Low back pain for 8 months

【Present Medical History】

Low back pain which becomes worse with exertion. Generally, this patient had a dislike of cold, cold extremities and copious urination. X-rays showed her to have retrograde degeneration of the lumbar vertebra.

【Examination】

Tenderness at L4 and L5. Lifting-leg test (+). Pale tongue with a white coating, thready pulse.

【Diagnosis】

Low back pain (due to kidney deficiency)

【Treatment Principles】

Strengthen the kidney, circulate channel qi

【Treatment】

BL 23 (*shèn shù*)	BL 25 (*dà cháng shù*)	BL 52 (*zhì shì*)
L2~5 *jiá jǐ* (EX-B2)		

Shù-point puncture (*Shù Cì* 俞刺) was applied. Cupping was done after needling. Treatment was given once a day. The pain was relieved after six treatments and cured after a total of 12.

【Note】

This is a patient with the retrograde degeneration of lumbar vertebra. BL 23 (*shèn shù*) was selected to tonify the kidney. BL 25 (*dà cháng shù*) to strengthen the lumbus and knees, and to regulate the channel qi in the lower back. BL 52 (*zhì shì*) is used to replenish kidney yin and strengthen the lumbus. *Jiá jǐ* (EX-B2) of second through fifth lumbar vertebrae, this is an important area for retrograde degeneration of lumbar vertebrae, it is punctured deeply to 1.5 inches directly into the transverse process of lumbar vertebra. Cupping is helpful in promoting blood circulation; it regulates the local channel qi. When the circulation of qi and blood

improves, the pain will stop.

> **Shu-point puncture** (*Shù Cì* 俞刺) *is one of the needling methods mentioned in The Yellow Emperor's Internal Classic. It says: "Shu-point puncture is when the needle is inserted deep as to the bone for treating the bony pain (Gǔ Bì 骨痹) which corresponds to kidney." This technique was developed in response to diseases associated with the kidney, the organ which controls the bones.*

Cheng Xin-nong's Medical Records

Li, male, 22, first visit was on September 1, 1992

【Chief Complaint】
Pain in the back and lumbar region for one week

【Present Medical History】
The pain started after exposure to wind post-sweating. The patient had a tense feeling in the back, aversion to wind, and was irritable, he had insomnia, yellow urine, and was constipated.

【Examination】
Tongue tip red, cracked in the middle, white dry coating, superficial tight pulse

【Diagnosis】
Low back pain (due to disharmony between *ying* - nutritive and *wei* - defensive)

【Treatment Principles】
Dispel wind and cold, regulate *ying* - nutritive and *wei* - defensive, remove obstruction of channels, stop pain.

【Treatment】

DU 14 (*dà zhuī*)	GB 20 (*fēng chí*)	DU 3 (*yāo yáng guān*)

SI 14 (*jiān wài shù*)	BL 23 (*shèn shù*)	LU 7 (*liè quē*)
LI 4 (*hé gǔ*)	PC 6 (*nèi guān*)	HT 7 (*shén mén*)
ST 36 (*zú sān lǐ*)	SP 6 (*sān yīn jiāo*)	LV 3 (*tài chōng*)
ST 44 (*nèi tíng*)		

DU 14 (*dà zhuī*), GB 20 (*fēng chí*), LI 4 (*hé gǔ*), LV 3 (*tài chōng*) and ST 44 (*nèi tíng*) were reduced. Other points, even method.

Four treatments cured him.

【Note】

The patient is constitutionally weak, his sweating is due to the disharmony between *ying* - nutritive and *wei* - defensive, thus allowing invasion of wind cold which obstructs the channels and collaterals of the low back, resulting in pain. The tense feeling in the back and aversion to wind are the signs of wind cold. The accompanying symptoms are the signs of heat, which is produced by the bottling up of qi by wind cold.

Li, male, 29, first visit was on December 24, 1992

【Chief Complaint】

Low back pain for two months

【Present Medical History】

The patient had a dull pain, which was sometimes worse and sometimes better, it radiated to the sacral region. Patient's urine was yellow and frequent.

【Examination】

Dark lusterless complexion, purplish tongue with tooth marks and a white coating, slippery pulse, proximal pulse weak.

【Diagnosis】

Low back pain (due to invasion of cold damp)

【Treatment Principles】

Tonify kidney qi, dispel cold damp, remove obstructions from the channels

【Treatment】

BL 23 (*shèn shù*)	DU 3 (*yāo yáng guān*)	DU 4 (*mìng mén*)
BL 54 (*zhì biān*)	BL 40 (*wěi zhōng*)	BL 58 (*fēi yáng*)
ST 36 (*zú sān lǐ*)	SP 6 (*sān yīn jiāo*)	KI 3 (*tài xī*)

Moxibustion was applied at BL 23 (*shèn shù*) and DU 3 (*yāo yáng guān*). A tonifying method was used at DU 4 (*mìng mén*), ST 36 (*zú sān lǐ*) and KI 3 (*tài xī*). An even method was adopted at other points.

The low back pain was greatly relieved after four treatments; all symptoms disappeared after 10 treatments.

【Note】

The kidney is located in the low back. When kidney qi is deficient, or cold damp invades, qi and blood will become obstructed, causing pain. The kidney controls urine and stools, its channel is externally-internally related with that of the urinary bladder. When the qi transformation of the urinary bladder is weak, there will be frequent urination.

Summary

Low back pain can be due to an invasion of external pathogenic wind cold damp, trauma due to sprain or contusion, as well as internal causes of damage to the kidney such as deficiency caused by excessive sexual activity, or overwork that consumes essence and qi. The lumbus houses the kidney. Problems with the kidney commonly cause low back pain; acupuncture is quite effective for this kind of low back pain.

Main points: BL 23 (*shèn shù*), DU 3 (*yāo yáng guān*), BL 40 (*wěi zhōng*).

GB 30 (*huán tiào*), BL 57 (*chéng shān*) and BL 60 (*kūn lún*) are added as symptomatic points for pain radiating to lower extremities. For those who have blood stasis due to injury from trauma, bleed BL 40 (*wěi zhōng*). DU 26 (*rén zhōng*) is added for stiffness and pain in spine and back.

STIFFNECK

Yang Yong-xuan's Medical Record

Wang, male, 33

【Chief Complaint】

Pain in the nape for 3 days

【Present Medical History】

The patient woke up with a stiff neck, it was seriously painful as he was unable to raise or turn his head.

【Examination】

Thin greasy coating, a slow lax pulse

【Diagnosis】

Stiffneck caused by an awkward sleeping posture (disturbance of qi and blood)

【Treatment Principles】

Dispel wind cold, warm the channels, remove obstructions from the channels

【Treatment】

LI 4 (*hé gŭ*)			
Right side:	BL 10 (*tiān zhù*)	GB 21 (*jiān jǐng*)	BL 12 (*fēng mén*)

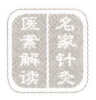

A draining method using a rotating motion was applied to BL 10 (*tiān zhù*), GB 21 (*jiān jǐng*) and BL 12 (*fēng mén*). A draining method using a lifting-thrusting motion was applied to LI 4 (*hé gŭ*). Moxibustion was used on GB 21 (*jiān jǐng*) after needling, and BL 12 (*fēng mén*) was cupped after needling.

One treatment cured him.

【Note】

The patient's neck pain was due to sleeping in an awkward position, this caused a disturbance in the local circulation of qi and blood, thus blocking the channels. For this treatment, local points and cupping are used together. The point *lào zhěn* (EX-HN19) needled with a draining method also can be useful. For serious pain, needle and drain BL 60 (*kūn lún*) and GB 39 (*xuán zhōng*), or LU 7 (*liè quē*) and *yǎng lǎo* (SI 6). These are distal points with good therapeutic effect.

> *Lào zhěn* (EX-HN19) is located on the dorsum of hand, between the second and third metacarpal bones, about 0.5 inch posterior to the metacarpophalangeal joint. Puncture perpendicularly or obliquely 0.5-1.0 inch. It is indicated for neck pain and pain in shoulder and arm.

Cheng Xin-nong's Medical Record

Liang, male, 34, first visit was on July 9, 1986

【Chief Complaint】

Pain on the left side of neck for two days

【Present Medical History】

Two days ago, the patient began to have a pain in the left side of the neck after reading a book for a long time at night. The pain was gradually getting worse, causing impaired movement. Although he had received both acupuncture and cupping, there was no improvement. Now, the pain was more severe and was accompanied by an impaired range of motion.

【Examination】

Local tenderness along the *taiyang* and *shaoyang* channels. Pale tongue, slightly yellow coating, deep and a bit slow pulse.

【Diagnosis】

Stiff neck caused by an awkward reading posture (obstruction of

channels and collaterals)

【Treatment Principles】

Invigorate the blood, remove blood stasis, calm the muscles

【Treatment】

Affected side:	BL 10 (*tiān zhù*)	SI 3 (*hòu xī*)	GB 20 (*fēng chí*)

Draining method. After acupuncture, the pain was gone and the neck could be moved freely

【Note】

The pain is located along the *taiyang* and *shaoyang* channels, thus points from the affected channels are selected for use. BL 10 (*tiān zhù*) and GB 20 (*fēng chí*) function to regulate qi and blood, remove obstructions from the channels and stop pain. The distal point SI 3 (*hòu xī*) is used to circulate the qi of the *taiyang* channel. The combination of local and distal points stops the pain by removing the obstruction of channels.

Summary

Stiffneck (*Lào Zhěn* 落枕) here refers to neck pain and motor impairment caused by sleeping or sitting in an awkward position and attack of wind cold that leads to disturbance of qi and blood in the channels. To effectively treat with acupuncture treatment the affected channels must clearly be sought out, and accordingly treated.

Main points: DU 14 (*dà zhuī*), BL 10 (*tiān zhù*), GB 39 (*jué gǔ*), SI 3 (*hòu xī*).

SI 14 (*jiān wài shù*) is added for pain in the shoulder or back, cupping can also be applied. BL 60 (*kūn lún*) added for difficulties in bending the head forward and backward, SI 7 (*zhī zhèng*) is used for difficulties in turning the head left and right.

CERVICAL SPONDYLOSIS

Yang Jia-san's Medical Records

Liu, female, 65, first visit was on April 4, 1987

【Chief Complaint】

Neck motor impairment with pain, a year ago the patient felt something snap in her neck

【Present Medical History】

This patient had impairment of movement with pain after feeling something snap in her neck, her right hand was numb, she had dizziness, headache, nausea, and a heavy sensation in her back which felt better with massage treatment, but was not cured.

【Examination】

There was pain whenever she moved her neck, although the range of movement was relatively normal. There was tenderness at C6 and C7. An x-ray examination showed abnormal cervical curvature, C4 to C7 hyperosteogeny, and narrowing of the intervertebral space. Impression: Cervical spondylosis. Tongue tip red, coating thin yellow, pulse deep wiry.

【Diagnosis】

Cervical spondylosis

【Treatment Principles】

Clear the upper, tonify the lower part

【Treatment】

GB 20 (*fēng chí*)	BL 10 (*tiān zhù*)	C4~7 *jiá jǐ* (EX-B2)
LU 7 (*liè quē*)	SI 3 (*hòu xī*)	

GB 20 (*fēng chí*) and BL 10 (*tiān zhù*) were drained with medium stimulation; even method with medium stimulation was for the rest of the points. The needles were retained for 20 minutes. Treatment was given once every other day. After ten treatments all the symptoms disappeared.

【Note】

GB 20 (*fēng chí*), BL 10 (*tiān zhù*) and cervical *jiá jǐ* (EX-B2) dispel wind and remove obstructions from channels and stop pain. LU 7 (*liè què*) connects with the *ren* vessel and SI 3 (*hòu xī*) with the *du* vessel; both of these extra channels originate from kidney. These two points used in combination regulate yin and yang, thus treating the root cause of cervical spondylosis and relieve pain.

Zhang, male, 80, first treatment was on February 23, 1987

【Chief Complaint】

Neck pain with range of motion impairment for three months

【Present Medical History】

Neck pain with range of impairment, numbness of hands, especially the right middle, ring and small fingers, occasional dizziness

【Examination】

Stiffness of the neck, pain appearing when the head is bent forward and backward, tenderness of the cervical spinous processes. X-ray examination finds a lack of cervical curvature, C4 to C7 hyperosteogeny, C4~C6 intervertebral stenosis, along with narrowing of the intervertebral foramen. Impression: Cervical spondylosis. Dark tongue with a yellow coating, deep slippery pulse.

【Diagnosis】

Cervical spondylosis

【Treatment Principles】

Clear the upper, tonify the lower

【Treatment】

GB 20 (fēng chí)	C4~6 jiá jǐ (EX-B2)	LU 7 (liè quē)
SI 3 (hòu xī)	SJ 5 (wài guān)	

These points were needled with medium stimulation once every other day. After treatments the neck pain was obviously reduced and after 10 acupuncture treatments it was completely gone.

Bo Zhi-yun's Medical Record

Xu, female, 55, first visit was on April 12, 1992

【Chief Complaint】
Impairment of range of motion in the neck, with tenderness for five years

【Present Medical History】
Impairment of range of motion in the neck along with tenderness, achy shoulder muscles, numbness of the left arm that radiated down to the ring and small fingers. The patient's sleep was disturbed due to numbness and pain of the hands, which is relieved to a slight degree with movement.

【Diagnosis】
Cervical spondylosis (due to spleen and kidney deficiency)

【Treatment Principles】
Tonify the spleen and kidney, remove obstructions from the channels

【Treatment】
Abdominal Heaven-Earth Acupuncture:

RN 12 (zhōng wǎn)	RN 4 (guān yuán)	KI 17 (shāng qū)
ST 24 (huá ròu mén)	the upper rheumatism point	

Twenty minutes after needling, the pain stopped and there was improved range of motion. On the following day, the patient reported that she slept without pain, and her neck had a more normal amount of movement when she awoke; the symptoms of pain in her shoulder and the left arm were improved by 70%. The same treatment was repeated seven times, after which all symptoms disappeared.

【Note】

Using the "turtle model" of abdominal acupuncture therapy, the location of points are in the shape a of turtle, which is seen as being a holo-image of whole body, with RN 12 (*zhōng wǎn*) as the turtle's head, RN 4 (*guān yuán*) is the tail, ST 24 (*huá ròu mén*) is seen as the shoulder, and KI 17 (*shāng qū*) located at the junction of the neck and shoulders.

The six points RN 12 (*zhōng wǎn*), RN 4 (*guān yuán*), KI 17 (*shāng qū*), ST 24 (*huá ròu mén*) are thus seen as a prescription for the treatment of cervical spondylosis. As it has something to do with the bones, cervical hyperosteogeny is related to kidney deficiency. Thus RN 4 (*guān yuán*) is used to tonify the kidney. While the incidence of cervical hyperosteogeny is rather high, only some patients have symptoms; most of them have some kind of functional problem with the cervical muscles. The spleen is the organ that dominates the muscles, so the spleen is tonified using RN 12 (*zhōng wǎn*). ST 24 (*huá ròu mén*) is used to circulate the channel qi of arm and head and KI 17 (*shāng qū*) is used as a local treatment. ·

Abdominal Heaven-Earth Acupuncture

This consists of the two points RN 12 (zhōng wǎn) and RN 4 (guān yuán). RN 12 (zhōng wǎn) is the Front-mù of stomach, it is externally/internally related to the spleen. The spleen and stomach are known as the Sea of Food Essence; RN 4 (guān yuán) also called Dān Tián, is the Front-mù of the small intestine. It functions to consolidate the kidney, reinforce qi and restore yang. They are used in combination with each other to tonify both the spleen and kidney.

Rheumatism points

These are Professor Bo's experiential points. The upper rheumatism point is located 0.5 inch supralateral to ST 24 (huá ròu mén), and the lower rheumatism point is located 0.5 inch infralateral to ST 26 (wài líng). They are good at relieving swelling and stopping

pain. Used together with SP 15 (dà héng) they function to dispel wind, lubricate the joints, and remove blood stasis. For treatment of the shoulder and elbow or the lower limbs, the corresponding upper or lower rheumatism points may be used singly.

Summary

Cervical spondylosis is a degenerative illness affecting the cervical spine that increases pressure on nerve roots, the spinal cord and the vertebral artery. According to Professor Yang Jia-san, the root cause of cervical spondylosis is liver and kidney deficiency leading to tendon and bone malnutrition. There can be concurrent invasion of external pathogenic wind cold that interrupts the smooth flow of qi and blood, or hyperactive liver yang causing *shaoyang* qi obstruction; in this case there is stiffness and pain in the neck along with dizziness. The development of this disease involves the post-heaven organs; the spleen and stomach. As there are symptoms of numbness, muscular atrophy, and spasm of sinews and muscles in the extremities. In this disease the pathological changes of the root (*Běn*本) are due to deficiency, while those of the branch (*Biāo*标) manifest as excess. Because the root is liver and kidney deficiency, while branch manifestation is in the head and neck. The treatment principles are to tonify the lower and clear the upper; points are mainly selected from the yang channels.

Basic points: GB 20 (*fēng chí*), BL 10 (*tiān zhù*), LU 7 (*liè quē*), SI 3 (*hòu xī*), and cervical *jiá jǐ* (EX-B2).

Supplementary points: DU 20 (*bǎi huì*) for dizziness. SJ 5 (*wài guān*) and *bā xié* (EX-UE9) are used to treat numbness of the fingers.

GB 20 (*fēng chí*) the intersection of the foot *shaoyang* gallbladder channel with *yangwei mai*, is excellent for dispelling both the disturbance from internal wind rising upward and the invasion of external wind. It is an important point for treating wind that is located in the nape of the neck; it is good for freeing up the cervical joints and improving the range of motion. BL 10 (*tiān zhù*) dispels wind cold and removes obstruction of the channels. As stated in the *Treatment of Diseases in Verse* (*Bǎi Zhèng Fù*, 百症赋):"Stiff neck with aversion to wind, BL 65 (*shù gǔ*) and BL 10 (*tiān zhù*) treats it."

LU 7 (*liè quē*) the *luò*-connecting point of the hand *taiyin* lung channel connecting with the *ren* vessel, it is used to diffuse the lung and dispel pathogens, regulate the *ren* vessel and treat pain of the neck and head. *Verse on the Four Most Commonly Used Points* (*Sì Zǒng Xuè Gē*, 四总穴歌) says: "For diseases of the head and neck, LU 7 (*liè quē*) is the most common point to select." The *ren* vessel pertains to the kidney, it controls the yin of the whole body, lung-metal produces kidney-water, reinforce the mother for a deficiency syndrome. Thus LU 7 (*liè què*) is also used to replenish the yin of the kidney. SI 3 (*hòu xī*) is the *shū*-stream of the hand *taiyang* small intestine channel, which connects with the *du* vessel. *Classic of Difficulties - The Sixty-eighth Difficulty* (*Nàn Jīng: Liù Shí Bā Nàn*, 难经·六十八难) says: "*Shū*-stream points are indicated when there is a heavy sensation in the body and painful joints." It is able to promote the circulation of qi in the channels of the back, and clear deficient heat from the upper *jiao* which subdues the disturbance of yang wind rising upward. The combination of LU 7 (*liè què*) and SI 3 (*hòu xī*) regulates both the *ren* and *du* vessels, which is to say, regulates yin and yang.

Cervical *jiá jǐ* (EX-B2) points, are located 0.5 inch lateral to the lower border of spinous process of cervical vertebra. Those between C3 to C7 are the most commonly used. Although not often found in formal textbooks, they are commonly used in clinic because of their good effect in removing obstructions from the channels and stopping pain.

In this prescription, GB 20 (*fēng chí*) and BL 10 (*tiān zhù*) are mainly used to treat the branch manifestation in that they unobstruct the channels and dispel pathogenic factors. LU 7 (*liè què*) and SI 3 (*hòu xī*) both treat in the branch by dispelling pathogenic factors and the root in that they tonify the lower, while clearing the upper, thus regulating yin and yang. *Jiá jǐ* (EX-B2) directly acts on the affected area by circulating qi and blood.

Xíng Bì (MIGRATORY ARTHRALGIA)

Lu Shou-yan's Medical Record

Wang, male, 22, first visit was on April 30, 1963

【Chief Complaint】
Migrating pain in the joints of the four extremities for two months

【Present Medical History】
A migrating pain, accompanied with range of motion impairment of the

knees and wrist, dizziness, listlessness, fullness in the chest, palpitations, and scanty yellow urine.

【Examination】

Swollen tongue, thin coating, wiry rapid pulse, pulse at GB 4 (*hán yàn*) is strong.

【Diagnosis】

Migratory arthralgia (*Xíng Bì* 行痹) (due to water weakness and wood hyperactivity, with floating yang wind)

【Treatment Principles】

Replenish yin, subdue yang, dispel wind, and transform dampness

【Treatment】

DU 20 (*bǎi huì*)	GB 20 (*fēng chí*)	DU 16 (*fēng fǔ*)
ST 35 (*dú bí*)	xī yǎn (EX-LE5)	SJ 3 (*zhōng zhǔ*)
LI 4 (*hé gǔ*)	GB 43 (*xiá xī*)	KI 3 (*tài xī*)
LV 3 (*tài chōng*)		

Tonifying and draining using both lifting-thrusting and rotating were applied.

KI 3 (*tài xī*) was tonified, the other points were drained; the needles were retained for 10 minutes.

After four treatments with the above method the dizziness and pain were reduced, however the palpitations and fullness in the chest were unchanged, the pulse remained thready, wiry, and slippery. The GB 4 (*hán yàn*) and ST 42 (*chōng yáng*) pulses were also strong. The pathogenic factor entered the heart, disturbing the mind. In addition to the previous method, treatment was added to calm the mind. Points: GB 20 (*fēng chí*), PC 4 (*xì mén*), HT 7 (*shén mén*), SJ 3 (*zhōng zhǔ*), LI 4 (*hé gǔ*), KI 3 (*tài xī*) and LV 3 (*tài chōng*). Tonifying and draining using lifting-thrusting and rotating were applied. KI 3 (*tài xī*) was tonified and the other points were drained; the needles were retained for 10 minutes.

After 12 acupuncture treatments, the pulse was a little wiry and rapid, the left side being bigger than the right, GB 4 (*hán yàn*) pulse was even. The tongue coating was thin white. GB 20 (*fēng chí*), PC 4 (*xì mén*), GB 4 (*hán yàn*), and LV 3 (*tài chōng*) were used to consolidate the effect, with the needles being retained for 10 minutes.

【Note】

Migratory arthralgia (*Xíng Bì*) is mainly due to invasion by pathogenic wind, and is characterized by constant movement and changes. This patient had an internal water deficiency leading to a wood hyperactivity, and then was invaded by wind cold damp. In this case the external wind and internal liver wind give rise to migrating pain, resulting in migratory arthralgia. His palpitations and chest fullness are due to the pathogen entering the heart. Professor Lu needled DU 20 (*bǎi huì*), GB 20 (*fēng chí*) and DU 16 (*fēng fǔ*) with draining technique to dispel wind and subdue yang. LI 4 (*hé gǔ*) and LV 3 (*tài chōng*), the four gates, were needled with a draining method to subdue yang wind. KI 3 (*tài xī*) was treated with a tonifying method to replenish kidney water thus softening liver wood. HT 7 (*shén mén*), PC 4 (*xì mén*) and PC 6 (*nèi guān*) were all treated with a draining method to remove pathogenic factors invading the heart. Additionally, local points running along the course of the affected channels are selected as local treatment to stop pain. Twelve treatments using this method achieved a remarkable effect.

Cheng Xin-nong's Medical Record

Shang, male, 65, first visit was on December 6, 1991

【Chief Complaint】

Migrating pain in the right arm for one week

【Present Medical History】

Pain radiated to the shoulder and back, the patient had dizziness, a slight numbness in the left cheek, and slept poorly.

【Examination】

Swollen purple tongue, thin yellow coating, and a thin, wiry pulse

【Diagnosis】

Migratory arthralgia (*Xíng Bì* 行痹) (due to weakness of the normal qi with invasion of pathogenic qi)

【Treatment Principles】

Dispel wind cold, remove obstructions from the channels

【Treatment】

GB 20 (*fēng chí*)		
Left side:	SI 18 (*quán liáo*)	ST 6 (*jiá chē*)
LI 15 (*jiān yú*)	SJ 14 (*jiān liáo*)	LI 11 (*qū chí*)
SJ 5 (*wài guān*)	LI 4 (*hé gǔ*)	SI 3 (*hòu xī*)

An even method was employed. After four acupuncture treatments the pain was relieved, after 10 treatments the patient was cured.

【Note】

This is a case of pathogenic wind cold and damp, with the wind being the most severe of the three pathogens, thus there is migrating pain. The dizziness, facial numbness, and poor sleep are the manifestations of qi and blood deficiency, which arise due to blockage of the channels and collaterals by pathogenic factors.

Zhuó Bì (DAMP ARTHRALGIA)

Lu Shou-yan's Medical Record

Chu, male, 30, first visit was on June 7, 1963

【Chief Complaint】

Extremity joint pain for many years

【Present Medical History】

Many years of extremity joint pain accompanied by numbness in the low back. Recently the patient had numbness and soreness in the right side extremities, the right hand was not able to grasp, along with soreness in the low back, seminal emissions, weakness in the lower extremities, dizziness, poor appetite, and loose stools twice a day.

【Examination】

Red tongue, greasy coating, *cun kou* pulse soft and a bit slow, KI 3 (*tài xī*), ST 42 (*chōng yáng*) and LV 3 (*tài chōng*) pulses thready, GB 4 (*hán yàn*) pulse big

【Diagnosis】

Damp arthralgia (*Zhuó Bì* 着痹) (due to spleen deficiency, damp retention)

【Treatment Principles】

Nourish water, inhibit wood, strengthen earth, transform damp

【Treatment】

GB 20 (*fēng chí*)	GB 4 (*hán yàn*)	KI 3 (*tài xī*)
LV 2 (*xíng jiān*)	BL 23 (*shèn shù*)	ST 36 (*zú sān lǐ*)
BL 20 (*pí shù*)	SP 9 (*yīn líng quán*)	
Right side:	LI 11 (*qū chí*)	LI 10 (*shǒu sān lǐ*)
GB 34 (*yáng líng quán*)	GB 39 (*jué gǔ*)	*bā xié* (EX-UE9)

Tonifying and draining methods of lifting-thrusting and rotating were applied.

KI 3 (*tài xī*), BL 23 (*shèn shù*), ST 36 (*zú sān lǐ*) and BL 20 (*pí shù*) were tonified, the others drained; needles were retained for 10 minutes.

【Note】

Damp arthralgia (*Zhuó Bì*) is mainly due to invasion by pathogenic damp, which is characterized by a feeling of heaviness. As the patient in this case has been invaded mainly by damp, there are manifestations of pain in the joints of the extremities, numbness and weakness in the low back and lower extremities, poor appetite and loose stools. Soreness in the low back and seminal emissions are signs of kidney deficiency. Dizziness and a red tongue plus the GB 4 (*hán yàn*) pulse being big means deficient yang is floating upward. This is a syndrome involving liver, spleen and kidney deficiency, where there is dampness together with liver yang hyperactivity. Moxibustion cannot be applied due to the deficient yang floating upward, so only acupuncture was used.

GB 20 (*fēng chí*) and GB 4 (*hán yàn*) are selected to clear the floating yang. KI 3 (*tài xī*), BL 23 (*shèn shù*), ST 36 (*zú sān lǐ*) and BL 20 (*pí shù*) are used to reinforce the spleen and kidney. LV 2 (*xíng jiān*) is needled to drain liver fire. SP 9 (*yīn líng quán*) is drained to transform dampness; points on the extremities of the right side are needled locally to remove obstructions from the channels and collaterals and to eliminate *Bì*.

Cheng Xin-nong's Medical Record

You, male, 26, first visit was on August 31, 1992

【Chief Complaint】

Pain with heaviness in both knees for half a year

【Present Medical History】

The patient states that his pain was due to invasion of wind cold. The pain was accompanied with heaviness in both knees. He also had epigastric distention and pain that was made worse by intake of cold food. Loose stools. Soreness in the low back.

【Examination】

Dark complexion, scalloped tongue with a white slippery coating, wiry,

slippery pulse, proximal pulse weak

【Diagnosis】

Damp arthralgia (*Zhuó Bì*) (due to cold damp invasion)

【Treatment Principles】

Dispel cold, eliminate damp, remove obstructions from the channels, stop pain, warm the stomach, strengthen the spleen

【Treatment】

GB 20 (*fēng chí*)	*xī yǎn* (EX-LE5)	ST 35 (*dú bí*)
hè dǐng (EX-LE2)	SP 9 (*yīn líng quán*)	GB 34 (*yáng líng quán*)
ST 36 (*zú sān lǐ*)	SP 6 (*sān yīn jiāo*)	GB 39 (*xuán zhōng*)
BL 60 (*kūn lún*)	ST 25 (*tiān shū*)	RN 12 (*zhōng wǎn*)
RN 4 (*guān yuán*)		

RN 12 (*zhōng wǎn*) and RN 4 (*guān yuán*) were treated with moxibustion. Other points were needled using an even method.

After 5 acupuncture treatments the pain in the knees and the distending pain in epigastrium were relieved. After 10 treatments, the distending pain in the epigastrium was greatly relieved and the heavy pain in the knees was gone.

【Note】

Invasion of cold and damp is the cause of the heavy pain in the knees. Cold damp damages the spleen, which dislikes dampness, leading to poor transport and transformation, resulting in distending epigastric pain and loose stools. The patient's dark complexion, low back pain, and proximal pulse weakness are signs of kidney deficiency.

Hè dǐng (EX-LE2), located in the depression of the midpoint of the superior patellar border, is indicated for knee pain, crane-knee syndrome (arthroncus of knee), and flaccidity of the lower limbs.

Tòng Bì (COLD ARTHRALGIA)

Cheng Xin-nong's Medical Records

Zhao, male, 23, first visit was on December 2, 1987

【Chief Complaint】

Pain in the left lower limb for three months, worse for about 20 days

【Present Medical History】

This patient's pain began three months ago after showering post sweating. About 20 days ago, after the weather turned cold, he began to have a pain in the posterior aspect of the left lower limb, which was worse at night and better for warmth, worse on exertion, and accompanied by muscle contractions of the lower limb. Herbal medication and over the counter anti-inflammatory medication did not relieve his pain. His appetite was mostly normal.

【Examination】

Purplish tongue with a white coating, wiry tight pulse

【Diagnosis】

Cold arthralgia (*Tòng Bì* 痛痹)

【Treatment Principles】

Remove obstructions from the channels and collaterals, invigorate the blood, and stop pain

【Treatment】

DU 20 (*bǎi huì*)	DU 14 (*dà zhuī*)	GB 20 (*fēng chí*)
DU 3 (*yāo yáng guān*)	BL 23 (*shèn shù*)	SP 6 (*sān yīn jiāo*)

Left side:	GB 30 (huán tiào)	BL 32 (cì liáo)
BL 40 (wěi zhōng)	BL 57 (chéng shān)	BL 60 (kūn lún)

GB 20 (fēng chí), DU 14 (dà zhuī), BL 40 (wěi zhōng) and BL 60 (kūn lún) were drained; other points were needled using an even method; moxibustion was applied to DU 3 (yāo yáng guān). Treatment was given once a day.

The patient came in with a serious pain and motor impairment of the left lower limb, by taking 4 OTC anti-inflammatory tablets he could sleep at night. Six acupuncture treatments, as outlined above, relieved his pain greatly. The motor impairment was basically cured. Without taking an analgesic, a slight pain still existed at night, but the muscle contracture of the lower limb had disappeared. His pulse was wiry and tongue light red. The same treatment was given 12 times in total, after which his symptoms stopped. He was asked to take special care, by not carrying heavy loads, and avoiding exposure to wind cold. Two months follow-up found no recurrence.

【Note】

Pathogenic wind cold damp, especially cold, easily invade when the pores are open after sweating and taking a shower. Thus cold arthralgia (Tòng Bì) is the result. For this reason, DU 14 (dà zhuī), GB 20 (fēng chí), and SP 6 (sān yīn jiāo) are used to dispel the pathogenic factors; local points are used to remove obstructions from the channels and collaterals. Even after being successfully treated, this patient needs to take good care in daily life, avoiding being attacked again.

Wang, female, 60, first visit was on March 1, 1993

【Chief Complaint】

Pain in the right upper limb for 2 months

【Present Medical History】

The patient reported the pain was caused by invasion of cold when she was feeling fatigued. It was worse in the shoulder and scapular region, and radiated to the elbow and thumb. She had problems with both abduction and lifting of the arm. The pain was better with warmth and made worse by cold. She had both fatigue and insomnia as well.

【Examination】

Pale complexion, emaciation, pale tongue with a white coating, deep and slippery pulse

【Diagnosis】

Cold arthralgia (*Tòng Bì*)

【Treatment Principles】

Dispel wind cold, eliminate damp, stop pain

【Treatment】

DU 14 (*dà zhuī*)	GB 20 (*fēng chí*)	SJ 5 (*wài guān*)
LI 4 (*hé gǔ*)		
Right side:	LI 15 (*jiān yú*)	*jiān nèi líng* (EX-UE12)
SI 9 (*jiān zhēn*)	SI 11 (*tiān zōng*)	LU 5 (*chǐ zé*)
SI 3 (*hòu xī*)		

Even method applied to all points.

After three treatments, the pain was relieved; she again had normal range of motion with her arm. Two more courses of treatment, although not continuous, were applied and she was cured.

【Note】

This patient had an invasion of wind cold damp due to a weakness of the *wei* qi. Cold is the most severe of the three pathogenic factors. Cold is characterized by contraction, thus the pain and impairment with the arm's range of motion.

Jiān nèi líng (EX-UE12) is located midway between the end of the anterior axillary fold and LI 15 (jiān yú) when the arm is hanging downward. It functions to dispel wind, remove obstructions from the channels and clear the collaterals. It is indicated for hemiplegia, shoulder pain with an inability to lift the arm, and pain in the medial aspect of upper arm. Method: needle perpendicularly 1~1.5 inches or needle through 2~3 inches to SI 9 (jiān zhēn).

Chen Yue-lai & Zheng Kui-shan's Medical Record

Xiao, female, 32, first visit was on December 5, 1999

【Chief Complaint】
Pain in the left lower limb for one month, worse in the past week

【Present Medical History】
One month ago, the patient suddenly felt a pulling pain in the left lower limb that extended from below the buttocks down to the dorsum of the foot along the posterior lateral side. Pain was made worse with walking, exposure to cold and fatigue. The hospital diagnosed her with sciatic neuritis and prescribed her Brufen and Fenbid. Bed rest and medication did not have much effect on her condition.

【Examination】
She had gait abnormalities as the toes of her left foot would touch the ground first when she was walking. There was tenderness at the spinous processes of lumbar vertebra (–), jaw-chest test (–), tenderness at the posterior aspect of thigh and the course of sciatica nerve (+), straight lifting leg test (+), CT showed no abnormality of lumbosacral vertebra. She had a red tongue with a thin white coating, and a wiry, thready pulse.

【Diagnosis】
Cold arthralgia (*Tòng Bì*) (due to cold damp retention)

【Treatment Principles】
Remove obstruction of channels and collaterals, stop pain

【Treatment】

BL 23 (*shèn shù*)	BL 54 (*zhì biān*)	BL 40 (*wěi zhōng*)

BL 60 (*kūn lún*)

Warm-opening method (*Wēn Tōng Fǎ* 温通法) was employed. BL 23 (*shèn shù*) was needled first and stimulated to cause a sensation to go to BL 54 (*zhì biān*) after which the needle was stimulated for one minute; then BL 54 (*zhì biān*) was needled causing the sensation to continue to travel down to BL 40 (*wěi zhōng*), it too was then stimulated for one minute; afterwards BL 40 (*wěi zhōng*) was needled causing the qi sensation to continue down to BL 60 (*kūn lún*), it was stimulated for one minute; finally BL 60 (*kūn lún*) was needled causing the sensation travel into the foot, again with another minute of stimulation. Needles were retained at each point for 20 minutes. Cone moxibustion was also applied. Treatment was given once a day.

After one treatment, the pain was greatly reduced. Three treatments completely stopped the symptoms.

【Note】

This is *Bì*-obstruction syndrome with cold damp retention in the channels and collaterals. Warm-opening method (*Wēn Tōng Fǎ*) is one of the traditional methods used to unobstruct the channels, in which the needling sensation is promoted and conducted to the affected area. Two techniques are used, one is to "urge the sensation" and the other to "connect it one point to the next". In this way, the channel qi or needling sensation is led along the affected channel in order to remove obstructions and circulate qi and blood.

Promoting the needling sensation along the channel to the diseased area includes four manipulations: Dragon swings the tail; here the needle is manipulated by swinging at a shallow level, Tiger shakes the head; this is where the needle is shaken at a deep level, Turtle drills the cave; here the needle is twisted with a drilling motion and Phoenix flies up and down; this is where the needle flies up and down by being lifted and thrusted. With this kind of manipulation, the circulation of qi and blood is promoted to remove the obstructions from the channels and collaterals. It is indicated for those syndromes of qi stagnation and blood stasis where patients with difficulties with feeling the arrival of qi, due to blockage of the channel qi.

Connect the needling sensation from one point to the next to the diseased area; like a relay race, the needling sensation is conducted from point to point on the affected channel to where the doctor wants the qi sensation to go. It is good in the treatment of hemiplegia, pain and *wěi-*flaccidity syndrome.

> *Dragon swings the tail*: a tonifying method of acupuncture. In manipulation, the tip of needle is pointed toward the diseased area, when the needling sensation appears, do not lift do not thrust, just swing the needle to both sides to strengthen the transmission of needling sensation to promote the propagation of the qi.

> *Tiger shakes the head*: a draining method of acupuncture. In manipulation, the supporting hand presses below the point to prevent the needling sensation from going downward, while the needling hand points the needle tip toward the diseased area. When the needling sensation appears, bend the needle body to the right so it looks like the letter "C", then bend to the other side, finally let the needle stand back up and give it a vigorous shake to spread the needling sensation along the channel.

> *Turtle drills the cave*: an even method of acupuncture. In manipulation, rotate the needle up and down, then left and right, while gradually thrusting it deeper and deeper; like a turtle drills the earth in all directions. Make the needling sensation appear repeatedly and transmit along the channel.

> *Phoenix flies up and down*: an even method of acupuncture. In manipulation, thrust the needle to the earth level first, wait for the qi, then lift it to the heaven level, when the qi comes under the needle shake the tail of the needle, then thrust the needle again to the human level, lift and thrust and rotate, after the needling sensation comes, quickly rotate the needle left and right while lifting and thrusting, rotate and release it repeatedly like a bird flying; make the needling sensation transmit along the channel.

Rè Bì (HEAT ARTHRALGIA)

Yang Yong-xuan's Medical Record

X X, female, 59

【Chief Complaint】

A burning pain in the left shoulder for two days

【Present Medical History】

One day ago the patient had a sudden fever and was restless, there was a burning pain in the left shoulder, difficultly in lifting the arm along with redness, swelling, and a hot sensation, accompanied by thirst and constipation.

【Examination】

Body temperature: 39.6℃ (103.2℉). Red tongue, peeled coating with cracks in the middle, slippery and rapid pulse.

【Diagnosis】

Heat arthralgia (*Rè Bì* 热痹) (due to consumption of yin and fire excess)

【Treatment Principles】

Clear heat, remove obstructions from the channels

【Treatment】

Left side:	LI 15 (*jiān yú*)	SJ 14 (*jiān liáo*)
LI 11 (*qū chí*)	SJ 5 (*wài guān*)	LI 4 (*hé gǔ*)

The ***Tonify First and Then Drain*** (*Yáng Zhōng Yǐn Yīn*, 阳中隐阴法) method was employed at LI 15 (*jiān yú*) and SJ 14 (*jiān liáo*); the draining method of lifting-thrusting was used at LI 11 (*qū chí*), SJ 5 (*wài guān*) and LI 4 (*hé gǔ*).

Herbal prescription:

川桂枝	chuān guì zhī	3g	Ramulus Cinnamomi
生石膏	shēng shí gāo	30g	Gypsum Fibrosum
知母	zhī mǔ	9g	Rhizoma Anemarrhenae
生山栀	shēng shān zhī	9g	Fructus Gardeniae (raw)
炒赤芍	chǎo chì sháo	9g	Radix Paeoniae Rubra (stir-baked)
淡子芩	dàn zǐ qín	6g	Radix Scutellariae
忍冬藤	rěn dōng téng	9g	Caulis Lonicerae Japonicae
忍冬花	rěn dōng huā	9g	Flos Lonicerae
制大黄	zhì dà huáng	6g	Radix Polygoni Multiflori Praeparata cum Succo Glycines Sotae (prepared)
生甘草	shēng gān cǎo	3g	Radix et Rhizoma Glycyrrhizae (raw)

One dose, in decoction form, taken orally

On the following day, the herb *jīn hú* (金斛) 9 g was added.

| 金斛 | jīn hú | 9g | Caulis Dendrobii |

On the third day, the patient's body temperature had lowered to 36.9℃ (98.2℉), the shoulder pain had improved, and the range of motion of shoulder joint had improved, the tongue was red, but showed signs of increasing moisture, thin and slippery pulse. Acupuncture and herbs were continued. She was treated for a total of five days, after which her shoulder pain disappeared and the movement became normal.

【Note】

Heat Arthralgia (*Rè Bì*) usually manifests with an abrupt onset of a burning pain in the joints and is accompanied by thirst and fullness in the chest. The patient here was treated with both acupuncture and herbs. This formula is a modification of *Bái Hǔ Jiā Guì Zhī Tāng* (*White Tiger Decoction Plus Cinnamon Twig*, 白虎加桂枝汤).

> **Tonify First and Then Drain** (*Yáng Zhōng Yǐn Yīn*, 阳中隐阴法):
> *Manipulate the needle at shallow and deep levels in the following way:*
> *The needle is first inserted to the shallow level and manipulated to tonify with a series of nine quick thrusts followed by slow lifts; then thrust to the deep level and manipulated to drain with six quick lifts and slow thrusts of the needle. It is used to treat disease that begins with cold and then turns to heat.*
>
> *This technique is opposite to Drain First and Then Tonify (Yīn Zhōng YǐnYáng, 阴中隐阳法). Both of them are indicated in complicated syndromes where there is a mixture of deficiency and excess.*

Record in *Acupuncture - Moxibustion for Difficult Diseases* (*Qí Nán Zá Bìng Zhēn Jiǔ Zhì Liáo*)

Zhao, male, 32, first treatment on April 6, 1983

【Chief Complaint】
Swelling and pain of the right index finger joints for one month

【Present Medical History】
Pain accompanying range of motion impairment. The erythrocyte sedimentation rate (ESR) was high.

【Examination】
Red tongue, thin yellow coating, rapid pulse

【Diagnosis】
Heat arthralgia (*Rè Bì*)

【Treatment Principles】
Clear heat, remove obstructions from the channels and collaterals

【Treatment】

Right side:	LI 3 (*sān jiān*)

The technique of ***Penetrating-heaven coolness*** was applied. The needle was manipulated once every five minutes and retained for 30 minutes.

After withdrawal of the needle, the redness and swelling disappeared and the finger could move freely. On the second visit, the pain basically stopped. One more treatment for consolidation was done and the patient was cured.

【Note】

This patient, who had signs of redness, swelling and burning pain of the joints, was diagnosed febrile *Bì*. The treatment focuses on treating the affected area with local points. As heat syndromes should be treated by clearing heat, the draining method is adopted to clear the pathogenic heat.

Summary

Bì means obstruction. ***Bì syndrome*** refers to those diseases characterized by pain, swelling and heaviness of muscles and joints caused by invasion of pathogenic wind, cold and damp which obstruct the channels and collaterals. If wind is the predominant pathogenic factor, migratory arthralgia (*Xíng Bì*) will manifest; if cold is predominant, the cold arthralgia (*Tòng Bì*) will be the outcome; should dampness be more prevalent, then the damp arthralgia (*Zhuó Bì*) will manifest. In prolonged cases, the various stagnations can transform to heat, with the associated presentations of heat arthralgia (*Rè Bì*) manifesting.

Removing the pathogenic factors from channels and collaterals is the principle for the treatment of *Bì* syndrome. Acupuncture is primarily used for migratory arthralgia (*Xíng Bì*); moxibustion with acupuncture is applied for cold arthralgia (*Tòng Bì*), and intradermal needling may be used in combination with other treatment for those with serious pain. Acupuncture and moxibustion are used to treat damp arthralgia (*Zhuó Bì*). Heat arthralgia (*Rè Bì*), is treated with acupuncture using a draining method.

The points along the *yang* channels in the affected area are selected and combined with distal points along the affected channels.

SI 3 (*hòu xī*), BL 62 (*shēn mài*), SP 21 (*dà bāo*) and BL 17 (*gé shù*) are chosen to treat pain anywhere in the body. DU 3 (*yāo yáng guān*) is used for pain in the low back. GB 30 (*huán tiào*), GB 29 (*jū liáo*) and GB 34 (*yáng líng quán*) treat iliac joint pain. *xī yǎn* (EX-LE5), ST 35 (*dú bí*), SP 9 (*yīn líng quán*), and GB 34 (*yáng líng quán*) are effective for knee joint pain. BL 57 (*chéng shān*) and BL 58 (*fēi yáng*) treat leg numbness and pain. ST 41 (*jiě xī*), GB 40 (*qiū xū*) and KI 3 (*tài xī*) are added for ankle pain. LI 15 (*jiān yú*), SJ 14 (*jiān liáo*), *jiān nèi líng* (EX-UE12) and LI 11 (*qū chí*) are used for shoulder joint pain. LI 11 (*qū chí*), LI 10 (*shǒu sān lǐ*) and SJ 10 (*tiān jǐng*) are selected for elbow joint pain. SJ 4 (*yáng chí*), LI 5 (*yáng xī*), SI 4 (*wàn gǔ*), SI 3 (*hòu xī*) and *ā shì* points treat wrist, palm and finger joint pain.

Use BL 11 (*dà zhù*) in cases of joint deformity; add BL 23 (*shèn shù*) and RN 4 (*guān yuán*) if cold is prevalent. Use BL 17 (*gé shù*) and SP 10 (*xuè hǎi*) in cases where wind is the significant pathogen. SP 6 (*sān yīn jiāo*) and SP 9 (*yīn líng quán*) are used for serious dampness. DU 14 (*dà zhuī*) is added to treat fever.

NUMBNESS OF THE EXTREMITIES

Yang Jie-bin's Medical Records

Ye, female, 24

〖Chief Complaint〗
Numbness of the fingers on the left hand for half a year

〖Present Medical History〗
The patient had numbness of the thumb which gradually after a few weeks involved the index, middle and ring fingers as well. Various biomedical examinations did not find any abnormalities. Muscular injections of vitamin B_1 and B_{12} and herbal decoctions were ineffective. In the past two months, the numbness became worse.

〖Examination〗
No swelling of the arms or fingers, skin colour normal, red tongue, thin white coating, thready pulse

【Diagnosis】

Numbness of the extremities (due to obstruction of channels and collaterals)

【Treatment Principles】

Remove obstruction to connect qi, invigorate the blood, and transform stasis

【Treatment】

LU 11 (*shào shāng*)	LI 1 (*shāng yáng*)	PC 9 (*zhōng chōng*)
LI 4 (*hé gǔ*)	LI 2 (*èr jiān*)	

Treatment was on the affected side only. The *jǐng*-well points were bled with a three edged needle; LI 4 (*hé gǔ*) and LI 3 (*sān jiān*) were drained. The patient was treated once every other day.

【Note】

The numbness is caused by the obstruction of channels and collaterals due to stagnant yang qi and poor blood circulation resulting in malnourishment of the muscles. The treatment principle is to remove the obstructions by opening the qi to improve the circulation of the blood. When the blood moves freely, the numbness will stop. Pricking *jǐng*-well points to cause bleeding promotes blood circulation and removes obstruction, thus improving the blood supply to the extremities. When this happens the numbness will naturally go away on its own.

Bo, female, 50, first visit was on October 28, 1978

【Chief Complaint】

Pain and numbness in both arms for 6 years

【Present Medical History】

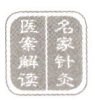

She began to have pain and numbness of the arms since November 1972, with numbness in the fingers and a cold pain in shoulder and neck. Four months ago her blood pressure was high. The treatment of western medicine was not effective, so she came for acupuncture.

【Diagnosis】

Rheumatic numbness of the extremities

【Treatment Principles】

Remove obstructions from the channels and collaterals, transform damp, and stop pain

【Treatment】

PC 9 (*zhōng chōng*)	LI 1 (*shāng yáng*)	SJ 1 (*guān chōng*)
LU 11 (*shào shāng*)	SI 14 (*jiān wài shù*)	BL 12 (*fēng mén*)

PC 9 (*zhōng chōng*), LI 1 (*shāng yáng*), SJ 1 (*guān chōng*) and LU 11 (*shào shāng*) were bled; SI 14 (*jiān wài shù*) and BL 12 (*fēng mén*) were bled and then cupped. After 10 treatments, she was basically cured.

【Note】

The patient lives in a damp place, and her constitution is weak, thus it was easy for wind cold damp to invade and obstruct the channels; stagnating the qi and blood. In prolonged cases of obstruction, bleeding directly removes pathogenic cold and damp. Once the obstruction is removed, the qi and blood circulation will improve, the pain and numbness will disappear on their own.

Summary

Má Mù (麻木), the numbness, known in ancient time as *Bù Rén* (不仁), is a subjective feeling on the part of the patient. Professor Yang Jie-bin holds that the pathological changes of qi and blood are the primary cause. Treatment should be based on the principles of removing obstructions from the channels and collaterals and regulating the flow of qi and blood. Based on his many years of clinical experience Professor Yang finds that bleeding the *jǐng*-well points is a powerful way to activate blood and transform stasis and connect with the channel qi. Other treatment is accordingly applied for symptomatic treatment. Then the channels and collaterals are unobstructed, and qi and blood flow evenly, the numbness of the extremities will be quickly relieved.

WĚI SYNDROME

Cheng Xin-nong's Medical Records

Hu, female, 21, first visit was on July 23, 1992

【Chief Complaint】

Non-growth of breasts for five to six years

【Present Medical History】

The patients' breasts were as flat as those of a little girl. She had a thorough gynecological examination in a local hospital, showing that she had normal hormone levels, a smaller than normal retroversion uterus, and a 2cm×3.5cm mass in the right lower abdomen. The patient thought of herself as being introverted and with a tendency not to express her feelings of anger. Her menses came when she was 15 and the menstrual flow was heavy and with clots, and accompanied by pain in lower abdomen and lumbosacral region. She had dizziness, fullness in chest, irritability, dream-disturbed sleep, and a poor appetite.

【Examination】

Sallow complexion, a mass in the right lower abdomen with a dull pain or no pain; purplish tongue, tip red, white coating, thready wiry pulse

【Diagnosis】

Wěi-mal-development syndrome (liver qi stagnation)

【Treatment Principles】

Calm the liver, regulate the flow of qi and blood

【Treatment】

| RN 17 (*dàn zhōng*) | ST 16 (*yīng chuāng*) | PC 1 (*tiān chí*) |

ST 18 (*rǔ gēn*)	LV 14 (*qī mén*)	RN 6 (*qì hǎi*)
ST 29 (*guī lái*)	PC 6 (*nèi guān*)	LI 4 (*hé gǔ*)
ST 36 (*zú sān lǐ*)	SP 6 (*sān yīn jiāo*)	LV 8 (*qū quán*)
GB 34 (*yáng líng quán*)	LV 3 (*tài chōng*)	

RN 6 (*qì hǎi*), ST 36 (*zú sān lǐ*) and SP 6 (*sān yīn jiāo*) were needled with a tonifying method, others were treated with an even method.

After eight treatments, her breasts and areola began to develop and the mass became smaller, her appetite improved, and she gradually gained some weight. With three courses of treatment, all symptoms were greatly relieved, her breasts became larger, and the mass was more indistinct when palpated. She did not continue the treatment as she lived very far away.

【Note】

This is a *wěi*-mal-development syndrome of breasts. The breasts and lower abdomen are areas nourished and influenced by the liver channel. The liver is like the General of an army; it likes order. Liver qi stagnation is the cause of her slow breast development. Qi disease involves the blood, thus the mass in the lower abdomen. When the liver overacts on the spleen, the production of qi and blood is impeded, thus the poor appetite and dizziness. Qi stagnation transforms into fire disturbing the heart/mind, thus irritability and insomnia. With qi stagnation and blood stasis, the liver fails to store blood and the spleen fails to control blood, thus the menstruation flow was clotted and heavy along with pain in the lower abdomen and lumbosacral region. The treatment principles are to calm the liver, circulate qi, and strengthen the spleen and stomach. The commonly used points are ST 18 (*rǔ gēn*), PC 1 (*tiān chí*), ST 16 (*yīng chuāng*), LV 14 (*qī mén*), RN 17 (*dàn zhōng*), LI 4 (*hé gǔ*), LV 3 (*tài chōng*), ST 36 (*zú sān lǐ*), SP 6 (*sān yīn jiāo*), SI 1 (*shào zé*), RN 12 (*zhōng wǎn*), and RN 6 (*qì hǎi*).

Wu, male, 43, first visit was on November 2, 1985

【Chief Complaint】

Muscular atrophy of the right leg for 20 years

【Present Medical History】

Twenty years ago the patient began to experience muscular atrophy in the right leg, now the thigh was beginning to atrophy too. The right leg was weak, the right side body felt cold, and sometimes there was a migrating pain. The right teeth felt weak when chewing. Walking was difficult. Appetite was mostly normal, as were urine and stools.

【Examination】

Muscular atrophy of the right leg; pale red tongue, with cracks in the middle and scalloped borders and a thin coating; wiry thready pulse

【Diagnosis】

Wěi-flaccidity syndrome (due to qi and blood deficiency)

【Treatment Principles】

Remove obstruction of channels and collaterals, strengthen spleen and stomach, nourish qi and blood.

【Treatment】

DU 20 (*bǎi huì*)	DU 14 (*dà zhuī*)	
Right side:	LI 15 (*jiān yú*)	SJ 14 (*jiān liáo*)
LI 11 (*qū chí*)	SJ 5 (*wài guān*)	GB 31 (*fēng shì*)
SP 9 (*yīn líng quán*)	GB 34 (*yáng líng quán*)	ST 36 (*zú sān lǐ*)
SP 6 (*sān yīn jiāo*)	LV 3 (*tài chōng*)	

ST 2 (*sì bái*) and SI 18 (*quán liáo*) were tapped gently with a plum blossom hammer; the foot *yangming* stomach channel on the leg was more aggressively treated.

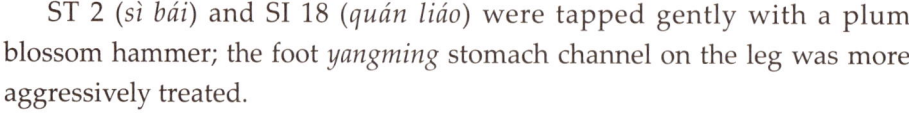

The above treatment was given 10 times, after which the symptoms were reduced. The tip of the tongue was red; the pulse was wiry. ST 6 (*jiá chē*), LI 4 (*hé gǔ*) and SI 3 (*hòu xī*) on the right side were added.

After more than 40 treatments, the right side of his body no longer felt cold, the strength of right arm was restored, but the right leg and ankle were still weak. So treatment was continued for another 15 sessions, after which the long-term weakness of the leg improved. Even though he had this muscular weakness for 20 years, 60 acupuncture treatments were still able to help relieve his condition.

【Note】

The ancient medical book says: "The *yangming* channel is the sea of five *zang* and six *fu* organs, it controls the moistening of the tendons, which bind to the bones and move the joints." This patient had a constitutional weakness of the spleen and stomach; prolonged illness further injured the qi of the middle *jiao*. The spleen and stomach's function of receiving food, transport and transformation were disordered, leading to qi and blood deficiency. The *zang-fu* organs, tendons, and bones lack nourishment, thus the impairment of movement in the joints and muscular weakness. To promote circulation of qi and blood, the plum blossom hammer is used to tap heavily on the foot *yangming* stomach channel of the leg and gently on ST 2 (*sì bái*) and SI 18 (*quán liáo*). In the *wěi* syndrome, the tendons and muscles are flaccid. The *yangming* channel is responsible for moistening the tendons. The liver dominates the tendons, but also involves the gallbladder due to their external/internal relationship. Thus, the points LI 15 (*jiān yú*), LI 11 (*qū chí*) and ST 36 (*zú sān lǐ*) of the *yangming* channel, SJ 14 (*jiān liáo*), SJ 5 (*wài guān*), GB 31 (*fēng shì*) and GB 34 (*yáng líng quán*) of the *shaoyang* channel, and LV 3 (*tài chōng*) of the liver channel are selected for treatment. ST 36 (*zú sān lǐ*), SP 6 (*sān yīn jiāo*) and SP 9 (*yīn líng quán*) are used together to strengthen the post-heaven nutritive aspect. GB 34 (*yáng líng quán*), the influential point of the sinews, is used to regulate the qi of channels to replenish qi and blood, which moistens and nourishes the tendons and bones. DU 20 (*bǎi huì*) and DU 14 (*dà zhuī*) are used to regulate yin and yang, and improve the circulation of qi and blood circulation. All of these points in this group function to remove obstructions from the channels and collaterals, strengthen the spleen and stomach, and replenish qi and blood.

Li, male, 14, first visit was on February 25, 1987

【Chief Complaint】

Muscular atrophy of the left limbs, hemiplegia for 13 years

【Present Medical History】

Since birth the patient could not open his right eye. Half a year later, it was discovered his left hand was unable to hold things, and his left leg was weak. Xuanwu Hospital diagnosed him with Congenital Infantile Paralysis. Injections of galanthamine and vitamins along with acupuncture did not improve his condition. This patient had impaired movement, intelligence was almost normal.

【Examination】

Ptosis of right eyelid, muscular atrophy of left limbs, red tongue with a thin white coating, deep pulse

【Diagnosis】

Wěi-flaccidity syndrome (due to liver and kidney essence and blood deficiency)

【Treatment Principles】

Replenish essence and marrow, remove obstruction from the channels, strengthen the tendons

【Treatment】

DU 20 (*bǎi huì*)	DU 14 (*dà zhuī*)	GB 20 (*fēng chí*)
LI 4 (*hé gǔ*)	ST 36 (*zú sān lǐ*)	LV 3 (*tài chōng*)
SP 6 (*sān yīn jiāo*)	GB 34 (*yáng líng quán*)	
Left side:	LI 15 (*jiān yú*)	LI 10 (*shǒu sān lǐ*)
SJ 5 (*wài guān*)	SI 3 (*hòu xī*)	LI 5 (*yáng xī*)
zhōng quán (EX UE3)		
Right side:	GB 14 (*yáng bái*)	GB 15 (*tóu lín qì*)

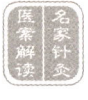

The hand *yangming* large intestine channel was tapped gently with a plum blossom hammer.

On May 15, 1987, after 60 treatments, the functions of his left hand were greatly improved, as were the muscles of the upper arm. The swelling of the left wrist went down and there was a reduction in pain. DU 20 (*bǎi huì*), DU 14 (*dà zhuī*), GB 20 (*fēng chí*), LI 4 (*hé gǔ*), LV 3 (*tài chōng*), SP 6 (*sān yīn jiāo*), and GB 34 (*yáng líng quán*). Right side: GB 14 (*yáng bái*), GB 15 (*tóu lín qì*), ST 2 (*sì bái*), and BL 2 (*cuán zhú*). Left side: LI 15 (*jiān yú*), SJ 14 (*jiān liáo*), LI 6 (*piān lì*), LI 10 (*shǒu sān lǐ*), LI 5 (*yáng xī*), and *zhōng quán* (EX-UE3). The large intestine channel of hand *yangming* was tapped gently with a plum blossom hammer.

On August 7, 1987, after five months of treatment, the movement of his left limbs, especially of fingers and wrist, was improved. The muscle of his left upper arm were also much improved. The ptosis of his right eyelid was better and the papebral fissure bigger. As he needed to return home for school, he continued treatment in the local hospital of his hometown.

【Note】

This patient has a congenital deficiency. There was a deficiency of liver blood and kidney essence, so the tendons, bones and muscles suffer a long-term lack of nourishment. Thus the appearance of muscular atrophy, which in Chinese medicine is referred to as *wěi*-flaccidity syndrome.

DU 20 (*bǎi huì*) the intersecting point of the yang channels regulates yin and yang, and promotes the flow of qi and blood. DU 14 (*dà zhuī*) disperses yang qi. LI 4 (*hé gǔ*) is a *yuán*-source point pertaining to yang; it controls qi. LV 3 (*tài chōng*) is a *yuán*-source point pertaining to yin; it influences blood. This combination, also known as the four-gates, harmonizes qi and blood and regulates yin and yang. LI 15 (*jiān yú*) is a point of *yangming* channel, which is believed full of qi and blood. SJ 5 (*wài guān*) is a *luò*-connecting point of the *sanjiao* channel of the hand *shaoyang*. SI 3 (*hòu xī*) is a point of the hand *taiyang* small intestine channel, which opens to the *du* vessel. This group of points unobstructs the channel qi of the upper limbs. ST 36 (*zú sān lǐ*) is the Lower *hé*-sea point of foot *yangming* stomach channel. SP 6 (*sān yīn jiāo*) is the intersection of the liver, spleen and kidney channels. This group strengthens the spleen and stomach, nourishes the liver and kidney, regulates qi and blood, and unobstructs the channels and collaterals. GB 34 (*yáng líng quán*) is the influential point of the sinews, it strengthens tendons and calms the liver. GB 14 (*yáng bái*) and GB 15 (*tóu lín qì*) are local points that circulate qi and blood.

> ***Zhōng quán*** (EX-UE3), *is located in the transverse crease on the dorsal carpus, in the depression on the radial side of the tendon of the musculus extensor digitorum. It is indicated for heat in the palm, abdominal distention and pain, cough and asthma.*

Bo Zhi-yun's Medical Record

Zhang, male, 11, first visit was on January 16, 1992

【Chief Complaint】

Motor impairment of both hands, weakness of the right lower limb for 11 years

【Present Medical History】

He was born after a difficult labour and suffered an intracranial hemorrhage due to the usage of obstetric forceps, which required a hospital stay of 52 days for treatment. Ever since birth, his thumbs flexed to palm, he was unable to extend them; the other four fingers could flex and extend, as a result his hands were useless. He was unable to take care of himself in daily life. His right lower leg was weak, the right foot dragged the ground when he walked; he often fell down.

【Diagnosis】

Wěi-flaccidity syndrome (due to spleen and kidney deficiency)

【Treatment Principles】

Tonify the spleen and kidney, unobstruct the channels

【Treatment】

Abdominal Heaven-Earth Acupuncture	ST 24 (*huá ròu mén*)

After five minutes of needling, the thumbs could stretch. After 30 minutes with retaining of needles, the thumbs could hold a pencil, but were not facile in movement. Two more treatments allowed his thumbs move much freely and he could eat by himself. The right foot was stronger when walking. He was asked to do some exercises as part of self care.

【Note】

Bo's Abdominal Acupuncture Therapy was used for this patient. The Heaven-Earth points are RN 12 (*zhōng wǎn*) and RN 4 (*guān yuán*), together they tonify the spleen and kidney. The kidney dominates bones and produces marrow. In case it is deficient, so the bones are weak. The spleen dominates the muscles and limbs. In this case it is deficient, so the limbs and muscles lack nourishment. Therefore, all the diseases related to spleen and kidney deficiency may be treated with the Abdominal Heaven-Earth acupuncture points.

Summary

Wěi syndrome is characterized by flaccidity and atrophy of the limbs with motor impairment. The causative factors are attributed to invasion of the lung by virulent heat pathogens, exhaustion of blood and body fluids, or the influence of heat pathogens which deprive the tendons and muscles of nourishment. This is seen in cases of acute myelitis, progressive myatrophy, myasthenia gravis, multiple neuritis, periodic paralysis, and so on.

The Ancient Medical Book says: "The *yangming* channel is the sea of five *zang* and six *fu* organs, it controls the moistening of the tendons, which bind to the bones and move the joints." "Points along the *yangming* channels are usually selected in the treatment of wěi syndrome." So, tapping the *yangming* channel with a plum blossom hammer is always part of the treatment; appropriate symptomatic points are needled as well.

PTOSIS

Zheng Kui-shan's Medical Records

Zeng, female, 7, first visit was on October, 2003

【Chief Complaint】

Ptosis of the right eye

【Present Medical History】

For no apparent reason this patient had ptosis of the right eye; the dropped eyelid covered half of her pupil, nor could she completely close her eye. She had additional symptoms of tearing when exposed to wind, excessive eye secretions, dry eyes, and blurred vision.

【Diagnosis】

Ptosis (due to spleen qi deficiency, with wind in the collaterals)

【Treatment Principles】

Dispel wind, remove obstructions, strengthen spleen, and tonify qi

【Treatment】

BL 2 (*cuán zhú*)	*tài yáng* (EX-HN5)	*yú yāo* (EX-HN4)
ST 2 (*sì bái*)	GB 20 (*fēng chí*)	ST 36 (*zú sān lǐ*)
BL 20 (*pí shù*)		

The warm reinforcing method was used. Treatment was given once a day, with 10 treatments constituting one course.

With two months of treatment, the symptoms were significantly reduced. She could blink and close the eye. Looking straight ahead, her eyes were basically symmetrical.

【Note】

Ptosis falls into the category of spleen qi deficiency accompanied by wind in the collaterals.

> *Warm tonifying method* is an acupuncture procedure created by Professor Zheng Kui-shan. The level of stimulation is somewhere between that of "Setting the mountain on fire" and "Inserting fire tonification". Clinically it is extensively used, with good results, for the treatment of deficiency cold syndromes. The method: the supporting thumb or index finger presses the point, the needle hand inserts the needle, after the qi arrives the supporting hand presses hard while the thumb of the needling hand rotates the needle forward continuously 3~5 times. After a heaviness and tightness come under the needle, press heavily and lift slowly for 3~5 times; the thumb then again rotates the needle forward 3~5 revolutions, while keeping the needle tip where the sensation is induced to cause the qi to remain there in order to promote the feeling of heaviness and tightness which will eventually produce a warm sensation. After retaining the needle, withdraw it slowly and press the point to close it. Treat once a day, 10 treatments constitutes one course. Depending on the case, treatment may also be given every other day.

Fu, female, 4 months, first visit was on April 2002

【Chief Complaint】

The mother reports her baby could not open the right eye

【Present Medical History】

The girl was born after a difficult labour. Since birth she could not open her right eye and blink. CT and MRI examinations showed no abnormalities. Injection of neostigmine provided a little relieve from the symptoms. It was thought that the levator muscle of upper eyelid was injured during the birth process.

【Family history】

No history of hereditary disease

【Examination】

Normal development, other than the inability to open the right eye, thus causing the pupil to be 3/4 being covered, eye movements were mostly normal.

【Diagnosis】

Ptosis (due to traumatic injury)

【Treatment Principles】

Remove obstruction of channels and collaterals, tonify the spleen to replenish qi

【Treatment】

BL 2 (*cuán zhú*)	*tài yáng* (EX-HN5)	*yú yāo* (EX-HN4)
ST 2 (*sì bái*)	GB 20 (*fēng chí*)	ST 36 (*zú sān lǐ*)
BL 20 (*pí shù*)		

The warm tonifying method was used. Treatment was given once a day, 10 treatments constituted one course.

Now, the child is 4 years old. Her right upper eyelid could be lifted to the upper border of pupil and she can blink freely, with no hypophasis. Eyesight: left 5.0, right 5.2.

Xiao Shao-qing's Medical Record

Cai, male, 27, First visit was on November 19, 1988

【Chief Complaint】

Ptosis of both eyes for 10 years

【Present Medical History】

Ten years ago, for no obvious reason, the patient suffered ptosis of both eyes, which was accompanied by hoarseness, lassitude of the loins and legs, which were better in the morning when he got up or after taking a rest, and worse after activity. The provincial hospital diagnosed him with myasthenia gravis. He was given pyridostigmine, potassium chloride and prednisone for 8 days as well as 10 doses of herbal medicine, he did not get any better, so he came for acupuncture.

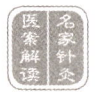

【**Examination**】

Ptosis of both eyes, difficulty in opening eyes; the pupils were covered. He had to raise his head and eyebrows, and frown to look at things. The tongue was pale with a thin white coating, and a thready, weak pulse.

【**Diagnosis**】

Ptosis (due to sinking of qi of middle *jiao*)

【**Treatment Principles**】

Strengthen the middle *jiao*, tonify the spleen qi, ascend the clear yang, tonify the kidney to consolidate the root, build up tendons and muscles, and open the throat to treat hoarseness

【**Treatment**】

Acupuncture and herbal decoction used in combination

①	*shàng míng* (EX-HN20)	GB 14 (*yáng bái*)	*yú yāo* (EX-HN4)
	RN 22 (*tiān tū*)	RN 6 (*qì hǎi*)	RN 4 (*guān yuán*)
	ST 36 (*zú sān lǐ*)	ST 43 (*xiàn gǔ*)	ST 44 (*nèi tíng*)
②	ST 1 (*chéng qì*)	ST 2 (*sì bái*)	GB 20 (*fēng chí*)
	DU 14 (*dà zhuī*)	DU 15 (*yǎ mén*)	RN 23 (*lián quán*)
	hǎi quán (EX-HN11)	HT 5 (*tōng lǐ*)	BL 23 (*shèn shù*)
	DU 4 (*mìng mén*)		

GB 14 (*yáng bái*) was needled through to *yú yāo* (EX-HN4). RN 23 (*lián quán*) was needled through to *hǎi quán* (EX-HN11), and BL 23 (*shèn shù*) was needled through to DU 4 (*mìng mén*).

The two groups of points were used in turns, once a day, with the needles retained for 30 minutes, 10 treatments was one course.

Herbal prescription: Modification of *Bǔ Zhōng Yì Qì Tāng* (Center Supplementing and *Qi* Boosting Decoction, 补中益气汤) and *Yòu Guī Wán* (Right Restoring Pill, 右归丸).

The ingredients:

黄芪	*huáng qí*	15g	Radix Astragali
党参	*dǎng shēn*	9g	Radix Codonopsis
当归	*dāng guī*	9g	Radix Angelicae Sinensis
炙甘草	*zhì gān cǎo*	5g	Radix et Rhizoma Glycyrrhizae Praeparata cum Melle
陈皮	*chén pí*	5g	Pericarpium Citri Reticulatae
升麻	*shēng má*	6g	Rhizoma Cimicifugae
柴胡	*chái hú*	6g	Radix Bupleuri
白术	*bái zhú*	10g	Rhizoma Atractylodis Macrocephalae
熟地	*shú dì*	6g	Radix Rehmanniae Praeparata
炒山药	*chǎo shān yào*	15g	Rhizoma Dioscoreae
枸杞子	*gǒu qǐ zǐ*	6g	Fructus Lycii
紫丹参	*zǐ dān shēn*	15g	Radix et Rhizoma Salviae Miltiorrhizae
杜仲	*dù zhòng*	8g	Cortex Eucommiae
肉桂	*ròu guì*	5g	Cortex Cinnamomi
制附片	*zhì fù piàn*	5g	Radix Aconiti Lateralis Praeparata
山茱萸	*shān zhū yú*	6g	Fructus Corni
鹿角胶	*lù jiǎo jiāo*	15g	Colla Cornus Cervi
肉苁蓉	*ròu cōng róng*	6g	Herba Cistanches
炒薏苡仁	*chǎo yì yǐ rén*	9g	Semen Coicis
补骨脂	*bǔ gǔ zhī*	6g	Fructus Psoralae
砂仁	*shā rén*	3g	Fructus Amomi

One dose each day. The herbs were decocted and the decoction taken three times a day.

After one course of treatment with acupuncture and herbs, the patient's appetite improved, and he was able to lift the eyelids higher, the hoarseness was relieved, and his loins and legs felt warm and stronger. After two courses, the muscles of the eyelids became stronger, and his speech clearer, and the loins and legs felt especially improved. A total of 30 acupuncture treatments and 28 doses of herbs were given, after which he was cured.

【Note】

The spleen controls the muscles. The upper eyelid pertains to the spleen. In the case of spleen qi deficiency, clear yang fails to ascend, or the wind obstructs the collaterals, causing ptosis. In differentiating the syndromes, there is spleen qi deficiency and wind affecting the collaterals. This patient suffers from spleen qi and kidney yang deficiency. The treatment principles are to strengthen the middle *jiao*, tonify spleen qi, ascend the clear yang, tonify the kidney to consolidate the root, build up tendons and muscles, and open the throat to treat hoarseness. In acupuncture, the local and distal points are used in combination.

Locally, BL 2 (*cuán zhú*), ST 2 (*sì bái*), GB 14 (*yáng bái*) needled to *yú yāo* (EX-HN4), *shàng míng* (EX-HN20) and ST 1 (*chéng qì*) are tonified to activate and regulate the qi of the foot *taiyang, yangming* and *shaoyang* channels, thus promoting the recovery of muscles and tendon function. RN 22 (*tiān tū*), DU 15 (*yǎ mén*), and RN 23 (*lián quán*) needled through to *hǎi quán* (EX-HN11), and HT 5 (*tōng lǐ*) are treated with an even method to open throat and treat hoarseness. RN 6 (*qì hǎi*), RN 4 (*guān yuán*), ST 36 (*zú sān lǐ*), ST 43 (*xiàn gǔ*), and ST 44 (*nèi tíng*) are used to strengthen the middle *jiao*, tonify the spleen qi, and ascend the clear yang. GB 20 (*fēng chí*) and DU 14 (*dà zhuī*) are used to bring the yang to the surface, which eliminates internal and external wind when treating diseases of the eye and head. Finally BL 23 (*shèn shù*) and DU 4 (*mìng mén*) are needled and treated with moxibustion to tonify the kidney, consolidate the root and strengthen the *mingmen* fire, thus supporting the spleen yang.

As for the herbs, *Bǔ Zhōng Yì Qì Tāng* (Center Supplementing and *Qi*

Boosting Decoction) aims at tonifying the middle *jiao* and replenishing qi to ascend the clear yang; *Yòu Guī Wán* (Right Restoring Pill) aims at replenishing essence and blood by tonifying kidney yang, thus strengthening the *mingmen* fire to promote spleen yang. In this way, the spleen qi is tonified, qi and blood are produced, and the function of the muscles in the eyelids can be restored.

Summary

Ptosis is a disease manifested as a partial or complete drooping of the upper eyelid due to problems with the levator muscle. In mild cases, a portion of pupil is covered; in severe cases, the entire pupil is hidden from view. This impedes vision, and is of asthetic concern to patients.

Congenital ptosis can occur on both sides or just on one side. As it is a heredity condition surgury is commonly used to correct the problem.

Acquired ptosis can be due to a variety of causes, it is divided into ① oculomotor nerve paralytic ptosis; ② sympathetic nerve paralytic ptosis; ③ muscular ptosis, often seen in those patients with myasthenia gravis, which is better in the morning, worse in the afternoon, and better with rest while but if continued for days it will quickly be aggravated again; ④ mechanical ptosis, caused by the weight of eyelid muscle, such as in cases of severe trachoma, eyelid tumor or hyperplasia; ⑤ others, like ptosis due to trauma, hysteric ptosis and so on.

Professor Zheng Kui-shan says ptosis is related to spleen and kidney pathology, because the former is the source of qi and blood and dominates the muscles, while the latter is the congenital root, storing essence and producing marrow, which nourishes the eyes. For the treatment of ptosis, acupuncture functions to strengthen the spleen and kidney, tonify the middle *jiao* and nourish qi, and remove obstruction of channels and collaterals. For infantile cases it is best to treat when they are 2~4 years old, as during that age they are less self-conscious about their image, while later this will be an issue.

Commonly used points: BL 1 (*jīng míng*), BL 2 (*cuán zhú*), *tài yáng* (EX-HN5), *yú yāo* (EX-HN4), ST 2 (*sì bái*), and GB 20 (*fēng chí*).

Supplementary points: DU 4 (*mìng mén*), SP 6 (*sān yīn jiāo*) and KI 3 (*tài xī*) are added for warming and reinforcing the kidney yang in the case of congenital kidney yang deficiency. ST 36 (*zú sān lǐ*), BL 20 (*pí shù*) and BL 21 (*wèi shù*) are added for tonifying the spleen qi in the case of spleen and stomach deficiency. SJ 5 (*wài guān*) and LI 4 (*hé gǔ*) are added to dispel wind and clear it from the collaterals of eyelid.

FACIAL SPASM

Cheng Xin-nong's Medical Record

Xu, female, 62, first visit was on August 3, 1992

【Chief Complaint】

Facial spasms on the right side for 10 years

【Present Medical History】

The patient reported her facial spasms were caused by exposure to wind after sweating and fatigue. She was treated in many hospitals for a number of years, but with no significant improvement. The exposure to wind, feeling nervous and fatigue would make it worse. The spasms were experienced by the patient as strong contractions, causing deviation of the eyes and mouth, and salivation during sleep. She had an aversion to wind and aching shoulders and back.

【Examination】

Dark complexion, frequent facial spasms on the right, pale tongue with toothmarks, white coating, and a thin, soft pulse

【Diagnosis】

Facial spasm (due to disharmony between *ying* - nutritive and *wei* - defensive, muscles lack of nourishment)

【Treatment Principles】

Dispel wind, harmonize *ying* - nutritive and *wei* - defensive, nourish qi and blood

【Treatment】

| DU 14 (*dà zhuī*) | RN 24 (*chéng jiāng*) | GB 20 (*fēng chí*) |

ST 2 (sì bái)	SI 18 (quán liáo)	SJ 5 (wài guān)
LI 4 (hé gǔ)	ST 36 (zú sān lǐ)	SP 6 (sān yīn jiāo)
Left side:	tài yáng (EX-HN5)	ST 3 (jù liáo)
	ST 4 (dì cāng)	ST 6 (jiá chē)

A tonifying method was adopted for the affected side, while a draining was used on the healthy side.

The frequency of the spasms was greatly reduced after eight treatments, as was the intensity of the contractions, the dark complexion also turned lighter. With continuation of treatment the spasms were further reduced to occasional episodes. Three courses of treatment brought her problem under control. A follow up three months later found no recurrence.

【Note】

The facial spasms were caused by an opportunitistic invasion of wind due to weakness of her exterior defenses as a result of a disharmony between *ying* - nutritive and *wei* - defensive. Wind is characterized by constant movement and rapid change, it has an upward and outward dispersion so it easily invades the upper part of the body; in this case the face resulting in spasm. This patient was constitutionally weak in qi and blood, so the muscles suffered a serious lack of nourishment; therefore the spasms were frequent and severe.

DU 14 (dà zhuī), GB 20 (fēng chí), SJ 5 (wài guān), LI 4 (hé gǔ) were selected to dispel pathological wind. PC 6 (nèi guān), ST 36 (zú sān lǐ), and SP 6 (sān yīn jiāo) were selected to harmonize the *ying* - nutritive and *wei* - defensive and nourish qi and blood. ST 2 (sì bái), SI 18 (quán liáo), tài yáng (EX-HN5), ST 3 (jù liáo), ST 4 (dì cāng), ST 6 (jiá chē), and RN 24 (chéng jiāng) were used for local symptomatic relief.

Yang Yong-xuan's Medical Record

Hu, female, 38

【Chief Complaint】

Facial spasm on the left side for seven years

【Present Medical History】

Irregular paroxysmal facial spasms. This patient tried all kinds of treatment, but without any improvement.

【Diagnosis】

Facial spasm

【Treatment】

Left side:	GB 20 (*fēng chí*)	*tài yáng* (EX-HN5)
SI 18 (*quán liáo*)	LI 19 (*kǒu hé liáo*)	BL 2 (*cuán zhú*)
Right side:	LU 7 (*liè quē*)	

The tonifying-draining Nine-Six method was used to treat this patient. LU 7 (*liè quē*) was tonified while the other points were reduced. The needles were retained for 20 minutes.

After more than 20 treatments her facial spasms gradually decreased and she was eventually cured.

【Note】

Professor Yang says that the facial region is a *yang* area. When liver wood is hyperactive it generates wind that moves upward and causes disturbances. As this is an excess condition a draining method should be adopted.

Summary

Facial spasms are manifested by irregular contractions of facial muscles on one side of the face. The causes are attributed to "liver wind", and sometimes fright. The defining characteristics are that it is mostly due to internal wind, and only occasionally caused by external wind invasion; deficiency syndromes are more prevalent, excess syndromes are more rarely seen. Onset usually is slow, but the problem can be intractable. According to Professor Cheng, the healthy side and affected side should be treated together, using fewer points with a tonifying technique on the affected side, and more points with a draining technique on the healthy side. The treatment strategy is to: a. nourish yin and blood, calm the liver to extinguish wind, b. harmonize *ying* - nutritive and *wei* - defensive, dispel wind, activate the collaterals, and c. harmonize qi and blood and calm the mind.

Commonly used points: DU 20 (*bǎi huì*), GB 20 (*fēng chí*), ST 2 (*sì bái*), SI 18 (*quán liáo*), ST 4 (*dì cāng*), ST 6 (*jiá chē*), SJ 5 (*wài guān*), LI 4 (*hé gǔ*), ST 36 (*zú sān lǐ*), and SP 6 (*sān yīn jiāo*).

To calm the the liver use SP 6 (*sān yīn jiāo*), KI 3 (*tài xī*) and LV 3 (*tài chōng*). DU 14 (*dà zhuī*), LI 11 (*qū chí*) and BL 12 (*fēng mén*) are added to dispel wind. To harmonize the *ying* - nutritive and *wei* - defensive add DU 14 (*dà zhuī*) and PC 6 (*nèi guān*). To calm the mind needle *sì shén cōng* (EX-HN1) and HT 7 (*shén mén*).

TREMOR

Cheng Xin-nong's Medical Records

Li, male, 37, first visit was on March 12, 1992

【Chief Complaint】
Tremor of the hands and feet for 10 years, worse in the past five years

【Present Medical History】
This patient had been treated in a hospital, but without significant improvement in his condition. He had obvious shaking in the morning when he got up, and a hot temper. He was unable to write, work or use chopsticks; slept poorly, was restless and forgetful. His urine was yellow, and at times he had bloody stools.

【Examination】
Dark complexion, red tipped tongue with a white coating, pulse was

wiry and slippery, the proximal position was weak.

【Diagnosis】

Tremor (due to yin blood deficiency, wind yang stirring)

【Treatment Principles】

Replenish yin to subdue yang, moisten tendons and muscles

【Treatment】

GB 20 (fēng chí)	LI 10 (shǒu sān lǐ)	LI 4 (hé gǔ)
PC 6 (nèi guān)	HT 7 (shén mén)	GB 34 (yáng líng quán)
ST 36 (zú sān lǐ)	SP 6 (sān yīn jiāo)	GB 39 (xuán zhōng)
KI 3 (tài xī)	LV 3 (tài chōng)	

GB 20 (fēng chí) and LV 3 (tài chōng) were treated by draining. ST 36 (zú sān lǐ), SP 6 (sān yīn jiāo) and KI 3 (tài xī) were tonified, all the other points were stimulated with an even method.

One course of treatment relieved the accompanying symptoms and five courses made a vast improvement in the tremors, as they only occurred occasionally.

【Note】

From the symptoms and pulse, the tremors were diagnosed as being due to yin blood deficiency, there was shaking because the tendons and muscles lacked nourishment. The restlessness and insomnia were due to disharmony between the heart and kidney with deficient fire. Fire disturbing the blood coupled with the yin deficiency gives rise to forgetfulness, yellow urine, and bloody stools. This is a syndrome of yin blood deficiency causing yang wind to stir; it is treated by nourishing yin and blood.

Zhao, male, 72, first visit was on June 30, 1992

【Chief Complaint】

Tremor of both hands for half a year

【Present Medical History】

The patient had yet to receive any treatment. The tremors were aggravated when he felt nervous. There was accompanying numbness of the fingers, poor appetite, dysuria, and constipation.

【Examination】

Dark complexion, red tongue with cracks and a white dry coating, wiry pulse

【Diagnosis】

Tremor (due to liver and kidney yang deficiency, leading to stirring of deficiency wind)

【Treatment Principles】

Tonify liver and kidney, moisten and nourish the tendons and bones

【Treatment】

GB 20 (*fēng chí*)	BL 18 (*gān shù*)	BL 23 (*shèn shù*)
LI 10 (*shǒu sān lǐ*)	PC 6 (*nèi guān*)	LI 4 (*hé gǔ*)
ST 36 (*zú sān lǐ*)	SP 6 (*sān yīn jiāo*)	GB 34 (*yáng líng quán*)
GB 39 (*xuán zhōng*)	KI 3 (*tài xī*)	LV 3 (*tài chōng*)

GB 20 (*fēng chí*) and LV 3 (*tài chōng*) were treated by draining. BL 18 (*gān shù*), BL 23 (*shèn shù*), ST 36 (*zú sān lǐ*), SP 6 (*sān yīn jiāo*) and KI 3 (*tài xī*) were tonified, the other points had an even method applied.

After one course of treatment the frequency and intensity of the tremors were reduced, and the fingers were no longer numb. Five courses of treatment cured him.

【Note】

This patient is elderly so has liver blood and kidney yin deficiency; the tendons and muscles are deprived of nourishment, which results in tremor of the hands and numbness of the fingers. The kidney qi deficiency and lack of body fluids moistening the intestines is the cause of dysuria and

constipation.

Summary

Tremor of the hands and feet, is a common condition in elderly people, it is seen more in males than females. It stems from liver blood and kidney yin and deficiency leading to a lack of nourishment of the tendons and muscles. "Yin relates to quietness, yang relates to movement." Nourishing yin and blood is the basic principle for treatment. ST 36 (*zú sān lǐ*) and LI 10 (*shǒu sān lǐ*) are the main points to accomplish this; symptomatic points can be accordingly selected, as can tonifying or draining stimulation.

LIVER WIND STIRING

Cheng Xin-nong's Medical Record

An, male, 7, first visit was on December 4, 1986

【Chief Complaint】
Restlessness and murmuring to himself for three years

【Present Medical History】
Three years ago, the boy started to be restless and murmur to himself. Before this he had a fever followed by convulsions. The children's hospital diagnosed him as being intellectually impaired and medicated him with Piracetam, but it was ineffective. At the time of his visit the boy was restless, murmuring, irritable, and unresponsive to questions. His sleep and appetite were mostly normal as were his urine and stools. He was a full-term birth, but his mother suffered from toxemia in the 8th month of pregnancy.

【Examination】
Red tongue, thin coating, deep thready pulse

【Diagnosis】

Liver wind stirring (due to kidney deficiency and liver hyperactivity)

【Treatment Principles】

Remove pathogenic factors, unobstruct the channels and collaterals, calm the mind

【Treatment】

DU 20 (*bǎi huì*)	*sì shén cōng* (EX-HN1)	DU 16 (*fēng fǔ*)
GB 20 (*fēng chí*)	DU 14 (*dà zhuī*)	RN 23 (*lián quán*)
PC 6 (*nèi guān*)	PC 7 (*dà líng*)	HT 7 (*shén mén*)
ST 36 (*zú sān lǐ*)	SP 6 (*sān yīn jiāo*)	SJ 5 (*wài guān*)
LI 4 (*hé gǔ*)	LV 3 (*tài chōng*)	

Acupuncture was performed without retaining the needles. After more than 20 treatments, he was much improved.

【Note】

This boy's previous febrile illness had not been completely resolved, lingering pathogens injured the liver yin, thus generating wind which disturbed the channels and collaterals, resulting in restlessness, and disturbing the mind resulting in his murmurs. DU 20 (*bǎi huì*) calms the liver, extinguishes wind and wakes the consciousness. *Sì shén cōng* (EX-HN1) calms the mind to promote intelligence. DU 16 (*fēng fǔ*) is a point on the *du* vessel that is influential in the treatment of wind; it scatters wind, opens the brain, and smoothes the circulation of qi. GB 20 (*fēng chí*) dispels wind and calms the liver. DU 14 (*dà zhuī*) settles the heart to calm the mind and to disperse yang qi. RN 23 (*lián quán*) clears the throat. PC 7 (*dà ling*), PC 6 (*nèi guān*) and HT 7 (*shén mén*) settle the heart and calm the mind. ST 36 (*zú sān lǐ*) and SP 6 (*sān yīn jiāo*) strengthen the spleen to promote intelligence and tonify the liver and kidney. SJ 5 (*wài guān*), the *luò*-connecting point and confluent point which accesses the extraordinary meridians, clears heat and unobstructs the collaterals. LI 4 (*hé gǔ*) and LV 3 (*tài chōng*), the Four-gates, calm the patient, calm the liver and extinguish wind.

> ***Toxemia of pregnancy***: *it refers to a critical condition that can appear after 20 weeks of pregnancy. It manifests as hypertension, edema and albuminuria; if serious it can result in convulsions, coma, heart failure, renal failure, even death of the mother and fetus. It is also harmful for the newly born baby, there may be delays in development, death, or premature birth.*

Summary

Although acupuncture is effective for **liver wind stirring**, the influence of family, school, and society all play a significant role in a child's development.

Main points: DU 20 (*bǎi huì*), DU 14 (*dà zhuī*), GB 20 (*fēng chí*), LI 4 (*hé gǔ*), and LV 3 (*tài chōng*).

Sì shén cōng (EX-HN1) can be used to treat intellectual disturbance. PC 6 (*nèi guān*), PC 7 (*dà líng*) and HT 7 (*shén mén*) are all good points for treating irritability. ST 36 (*zú sān lǐ*) and SP 6 (*sān yīn jiāo*) are good for improving the weak constitution.

EPILEPSY

Yang Jia-san's Medical Record

Wei, female, 12, first visit was on September 28, 1992

【Chief Complaint】

Epilepsy for six years

【Present Medical History】

The patient was hot tempered. She began having epileptic attacks at the age of 6. They would occur at least once daily and sometimes five to six episodes in a single day. When having a mild attack, she would stare mindlessly for a number of seconds and then come back. When having a serious attack there would be convulsions, which started from her mouth or finger, and would quickly involve her upper limbs or half her body. An EEG showed a serious epilepsy wave, thus the diagnosis of epilepsy. Medication did not prove to be effective. She had a poor appetite, ground her teeth while sleeping, was constipated and would pass dry stool like that of a sheep once every three to four days, urination was normal.

【Anamnesis】

The patient experienced oxygen deprivation while being born

【Examination】

Dull expression in the eyes and upon the face. MRI showed an uneven distribution of grey matter on the left side in the occipital parietal region. Red tongue with a slightly greasy, yellow coating, and a wiry and slippery pulse.

【Diagnosis】

Epilepsy (due to wind phlegm brought up by counterflow qi)

【Treatment Principles】

Extinguish wind, transform phlegm, calm the mind, and stabilize the will

【Treatment】

DU 14 (dà zhuī)	GB 20 (fēng chí)	GB 13 (běn shén)
DU 24 (shén tíng)	sì shén cōng (EX-HN1)	ST 25 (tiān shū)
RN 12 (zhōng wǎn)	RN 6 (qì hǎi)	SJ 5 (wài guān)
GB 41 (zú lín qì)		

RN 6 (qì hǎi) was treated with an even method. The other points were drained. SJ 5 (wài guān) was needled through to PC 6 (nèi guān). GB 20 (fēng chí) was needled toward the tip of the nose to a depth of 0.5~0.9 inches without retaining the needle. DU 14 (dà zhuī) was needled perpendicularly

0.8~1.2 inches without retaining the needle. GB 13 (*běn shén*), DU 24 (*shén tíng*) and *sì shén cōng* (EX-HN1) were needled obliquely 0.3 inch to the subcutaneous level.

The above-mentioned treatment was applied once every other day with the needles being retained for 30 minutes. She did not have attack till October 9, 1992, but when she did the convulsions suddenly started from the mouth and spread to the limbs while she waited for treatment in the waiting-room. She was quickly carried to the treatment table and treated at DU 26 (*rén zhōng*), LI 4 (*hé gǔ*), LV 3 (*tài chōng*), SI 3 (*hòu xī*) and BL 62 (*shēn mài*). Ten minutes later she came to. After a short rest, she was treated again with the previous points. During lunch that day, she had another attack after feeling crabby. Afterwards her seizures stopped, her emotional state improved, she had more liveliness in her eyes and her temper was more even, additionally her body became physically stronger as her appetite improved, she slept better and her bowel movements were normal.

An EEG examination on January 7, 1993, compared with the EEG taken on September 25, 1992, showed a great improvement. Acupuncture was continued and the dosage of medicine she was taking was reduced and finally stopped.

【Note】

According to Professor Yang, epilepsy is mainly due to wind, phlegm, and counterflow qi. During the attack DU 26 (*rén zhōng*), KI 1 (*yǒng quán*), DU 20 (*bǎi huì*), LI 4 (*hé gǔ*) and LV 3 (*tài chōng*) should be selected. Add SI 3 (*hòu xī*) and BL 62 (*shēn mài*) to open the orifices, wake the consciousness and stop convulsions. Between episodes the treatment strategy is to extinguish wind, transform phlegm, and calm the mind, in other words; treat the root i.e. wind and phlegm.

SJ 5 (*wài guān*), the *luò*-connecting point of the *sanjiao* channel of the hand *shaoyang*, is indicated in diseases of disordered qi; it regulates qi and transforms phlegm, when needled through to PC 6 (*nèi guān*) it treats mental disorders. GB 41 (*zú lín qì*) calms the liver, extinguishes wind, and transforms phlegm. These two are paired confluent points and thus work synergistically in calming the liver, extinguishing wind, regulating qi, and transforming phlegm; they are primary points in the treatment of epilepsy. GB 20 (*fēng chí*) is an important point for treating wind. DU 14 (*dà zhuī*) is a point on the *du* vessel that goes directly into the brain, it functions to calm the mind and settle the will. As wind is a yang pathogenic factor that easily transforms into heat, DU 14 (*dà zhuī*) is useful for clearing heat as well.

DU 24 (*shén tíng*) is an intersecting point of the *du* vessel with the foot *taiyang* bladder channel; GB 13 (*běn shén*) is a crossing point of the foot *shaoyang* gallbladder channel and the *yangwei mai*, these points are drained to treat the wind, fire and phlegm of the *shaoyang* channel that manifests as epilepsy with foamy phlegm on the lips during an attack. *Sì shén cōng* (EX-HN1) is an effective point for calming the mind and settling the will. The spleen is said to be the source of phlegm, the spleen and stomach have an interior/exterior relationship, so RN 12 (*zhōng wǎn*), the Front-*mù* of the stomach, is treated to transform phlegm. ST 25 (*tiān shū*), the Front-*mù* of the large intestine, is used to unobstruct the intestine that must be open to successfully treat the stomach. RN 6 (*qì hǎi*), the sea of qi, is used to regulate qi and transform phlegm. These four points are also called the four gates; they regulate qi, transform phlegm, strengthen the spleen and harmonize the stomach.

Cheng Xin-nong's Medical Record

Yu, male, 35, first visit was on November 7, 1986

【Chief Complaint】
Intermittent disturbance of consciousness for 16 years

【Present Medical History】
Sixteen years ago during the Cultural Revolution, this patient was sent down to the countryside to work on the farms. There he had some experiences that put a fright into him; he would have episodes where he would stare blankly and be incommunicative for 5~10 minutes. The EEG showed the presence of an epilepsy wave. At the time of his visit, he was taking luminal and diazepam everyday. He would have six to seven attacks

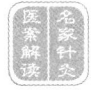

each month. When the attack was about to start, his complexion would turn yellowish blue, his limbs became weak, or he would have a coughing fit that turned his face red. During the attack, he turned pale, lips were purple, he would stare uncomprehendingly, sometimes foam at the mouth; his right limbs would stiffen and convulse, and sometimes he lost bladder control. This patient was generally irritable and irascible. He had coughing with profuse sputum that was difficult to expectorate, uncoordinated movement, poor appetite, poor sleep, abdominal distension and gas, dry mouth with preference for hot drinks, dry stools, and yellow urine.

【Anamnesis】

He was born after a difficult labour in which he suffered neonatal asphyxia

【Examination】

Swollen pale tongue with a thin slightly greasy coating, and a deep, thready wiry pulse

【Diagnosis】

Epilepsy (qi stagnation, phlegm retention)

【Treatment Principles】

Regulate qi, transform phlegm, augment qi and blood

【Treatment】

DU 20 (bǎi huì)	sì shén cōng (EX-HN1)	GB 20 (fēng chí)
RN 4 (guān yuán)	SI 3 (hòu xī)	HT 7 (shén mén)
ST 36 (zú sān lǐ)	ST 40 (fēng lóng)	BL 62 (shēn mài)
SP 6 (sān yīn jiāo)	LV 3 (tài chōng)	KI 3 (tài xī)

An even method was applied to all points. After 30 treatments his condition showed signs of improvement.

【Note】

This patient's epilepsy was caused by fright that disordered the qi.

As a result the body fluids are not properly transported along their usual pathways and turn to phlegm, which blocks the channels and collaterals. Failure of qi and blood to nourish leads to the pale complexion and purple lips. The uncomprehending staring, and seizures are due to poor nourishment of the brain. Prolonged disease results in deficiency of qi and blood, this is reflected in the pale complexion, pale tongue, and deep thready pulse. Liver stagnation, failing to maintain the free flow of qi affects the spleen earth, so there are signs of belching, abdominal distention, and poor appetite. This is an example of qi and blood deficiency with qi stagnation and phlegm retention.

Summary

Epilepsy, known as *Yáng Xián Fēng* (羊痫风), is characterized by the occurrence of seizures which can range from grand mal to petit mal to focal or psychomotor seizures. The grand mal epilepsy is manifested by fits where the patient falls down and loses consciousness, they may scream or simply stare, staring upward, frequently with accompanying convulsions. All of which passes after a few minutes and the patient's consciousness returns to normal. The petit mal epilepsy is characterized by only a momentary loss of attention with eyes staring blankly, but no convulsions. The principle for treatment is to open the orifices, transform phlegm, calm the liver, and extinguish the wind.

During seizures: DU 20 (*bǎi huì*), DU 26 (*rén zhōng*), and LI 4 (*hé gǔ*) needled through to PC 8 (*láo gōng*).

In between seizures: DU 20 (*bǎi huì*), GB 20 (*fēng chí*), DU 14 (*dà zhuī*), DU 8 (*jīn suō*), PC 5 (*jiān shǐ*), and *yāo qí* (EX-B9).

Grand mal epilepsy: daytime seizure: add BL 62 (*shēn mài*); night seizure: add KI 6 (*zhào hǎi*).

Petit mal epilepsy: add HT 7 (*shén mén*), PC 6 (*nèi guān*), and *yìn táng* (EX-HN3).

Focal seizure: add LI 4 (*hé gǔ*), LV 3 (*tài chōng*), and GB 34 (*yáng líng quán*).

Yāo qí (EX-B9) is 2 inches directly above the tip of coccyx, in the depression between the sacral horns. It is indicated for use in combination with DU 14 (*dà zhuī*) and DU 20 (*bǎi huì*) for epilepsy. The insertion of needle is subcutaneous and pointing upward along the du vessel 2~3 inches.

HYSTERIA

Record in *Acupuncture - Moxibustion for Difficult Diseases* (*Qí Nán Zá Bìng Zhēn Jiŭ Zhì Liáo*)

Fang, female, 27, first visit was on June 9, 1986

【**Chief Complaint**】

Inappropriate laughing and crying, occasional convulsions of the four limbs for four years

【**Present Medical History**】

This patient had inappropriate episodes of laughter and crying, and occasional convulsions of the four limbs, there was also a year by year decline in her memory. The previous treatment, which included both modern medicine and Chinese medicine, was not effective, and her condition was gradually declining. From May of 1986, it became worse. Yesterday she had more than 10 hysteria attacks during the day, and it was worse at night.

【**Examination**】

Pale tongue, thin coating, thready pulse

【**Diagnosis**】

Hysteria

【**Treatment**】

DU 24 (*shén tíng*)

Lifting method (*Chōu Qì Fǎ* 抽气法) was applied. This is a needling technique where the point is stimulated with a violent and rapid motion, with the needle then being retained for 48 hours or more. The patient is then taught a deep thoughtful breathing technique that focuses on drawing the breath into the abdomen, as a way to get them to relax.

After needling, the symptoms stopped. During the three days the needle was retained she only had two hysterical episodes.

【Note】

This patient's hysteria can be seen as a kind of epileptic seizure. DU 24 (*shén tíng*), a point on the *du* vessel, functions to treat headache, epilepsy, and rhinorrhea with turbid discharge. In the treatment for different diseases, different methods of manipulation should be adopted; supplementary thought-breathing exercises can also be given.

> ***Lifting-Thrusting method*** *(Chōu Tiān Fǎ 抽添法), includes the Lifting method (Chōu Qì Fǎ 抽气法) and Thrusting method (Tiān Qì Fǎ 添气法), it is a compound technique of lifting thrusting that can be used to both tonify or drain.*
>
> ***Lifting method*** *(Chōu Qì Fǎ) is draining while the Thrusting method (Tiān Qì Fǎ) is tonifying. The needle is retained from 2~24 hours, and even up to 24~48 hours. During this time the needle is manipulated once or twice. The lifting method (Chōu Qì Fǎ) in the scalp acupuncture is done in this way: after routine disinfection, a 1.5 inch filiform needle, 30 or 32 gauge, is inserted at a 15° angle toward the lower level of galea aponeurotica, thrust slowly horizontally about one inch, and then lifted three times with a strong break-out force. The needle body is not moved or only moved 0.1 inch, and thrust slowly about one inch again. Repeat the lifting and thrusting till the arrival of qi. **Thrusting method** (Tiān Qì Fǎ) is done with the manipulation of the needle in the opposite way.*

> ***Scalp acupuncture plus thought-breathing exercises*** *(Tǒu Zhēn Dǎo Yǐn Fǎ 头针导引法) includes both active and passive exercises. In the active exercise, the doctor and the patient both do Yì Niàn-thought and body movement. Yì Niàn-thought treats the Shén-spirit. While the needle is being manipulated, the doctor asks the patient to do Yì Niàn-thought by concentrating on the affected area. Yì Niàn-thought brings the movement to the affected area. Yì Niàn-thought and the body movement should be in combination with each other. Yì Niàn-thought has two functions. One is to activate and conduct channel qi to the affected area, the other is to lead the pathogen out. The passive exercise is for those who are unable to move the healthy limb, or need other people to help the affected side to move. For instance, for the patient with urine retention, during manipulating and retaining of the needle, when he does abdominal breathing, the doctor or a family member presses the lower abdomen*

toward the urethra; for the patient with hemiplegia, the doctor helps him to sit up repeatedly and walk. Those who are unable to sit should flex the knees, stretch the legs, flex the elbows, and stretch the arms in bed.

Cheng Xin-nong's Medical Record

Xi, male, 18, first visit was on November 16, 1987

【Chief Complaint】

Unable to speak for one day

【Present Medical History】

Yesterday at about 11 o'clock, for no apparent reason the patient was suddenly unable to speak; he lost his way home and someone had to bring him back. He had tetany and aphasia when he was seven. He was treated by Professor Cheng, and got better and could do physical labour. There has not been any reoccurrence for more than 10 years. At the time of his visit with the exception of being, unable to speak, his sleep and appetite were good and urine and stools were normal.

【Examination】

Dull eyes, red tongue with a thin white coating, thready rapid pulse

【Diagnosis】

Hysteric aphasia (due to heart and spleen deficiency)

【Treatment Principles】

Regulate qi and blood, open that which is closed, open the orifices

【Treatment】

DU 20 (*bǎi huì*)	DU 14 (*dà zhuī*)	RN 23 (*lián quán*)
LI 4 (*hé gǔ*)	SP 6 (*sān yīn jiāo*)	LU 7 (*liè quē*)
KI 6 (*zhào hǎi*)	LV 3 (*tài chōng*)	

RN 23 (*lián quán*) was needled without retention of the needle. Others were treated with an even method.

In the afternoon, after the treatment, he could again speak. Another four acupuncture treatments were done for consolidation using DU 20 (*bǎi huì*), RN 23 (*lián quán*) (no retaining), LI 4 (*hé gǔ*), LU 7 (*liè quē*), KI 6 (*zhào hǎi*), and LV 3 (*tài chōng*).

【Note】

As a child he had tetany due to deficiency-wind disturbance. Now his yin and blood were depleted, thus depriving the channels of nourishment, thus his mouth was blocked and he was unable to speak. The *shén*-mind was lacking nourishment, so the eyes were dull.

DU 20 (*bǎi huì*) opens the orifices and opens that which is closed. DU 14 (*dà zhuī*) calms the mind and disperses yang qi. RN 23 (*lián quán*) is the local point for aphasia. LU 7 (*liè quē*), of the lung channel, connects to the *ren* vessel which ascends to the throat. KI 6 (*zhào hǎi*) connects to the *yinqiao mai* which also ascends to the throat. The combination of these two points opens the throat to allow speech. TCM holds that kidney is the root of speech and lung the door of the voice. These two points are effective to treat aphasia and hoarseness. LI 4 (*hé gǔ*), SP 6 (*sān yīn jiāo*) and LV 3 (*tài chōng*) are used to regulate qi and blood.

Summary

Hysteria is a kind of neurosis. TCM holds that it is usually caused by emotional depression and over-thinking. The patient has sudden onset of psycho-emotive symptoms that could include violent behaviour, laughing and crying, sleeping all the time, or dysphonia, limb paralysis, epileptic like trembling and spasms, or sudden loss of hearing and vision, all without organic pathological changes which could be found in bio-medical examinations. Acupuncture may be applied together with suggestion therapy.

Main points: DU 26 (*rén zhōng*), PC 6 (*nèi guān*), HT 7 (*shén mén*).

LI 4 (*hé gǔ*) and LV 3 (*tài chōng*) are added for epileptic cases. DU 15 (*yǎ mén*), GB 30 (*huán tiào*) and GB 34 (*yáng líng quán*) are added for paralysis. PC 7 (*dà líng*) and KI 1 (*yǒng quán*) can be needled for sleeping all the time. RN 22 (*tiān tū*) is added for globus hystericus. BL 1 (*jīng míng*) can be used for loss of vision. SI 19 (*tīng gōng*) and SJ 17 (*yì fēng*) are added for loss of hearing. RN 23 (*lián quán*) and HT 5 (*tōng lǐ*) are added for inability to speak.

MELANCHOLIA

Cheng Xin-nong's Medical Records

Zhang, female, 21, first visit was on September 27, 1984

【Chief Complaint】

A sensation of something in the throat for one year

【Present Medical History】

One year ago, the patient began to feel a blockage in her throat and an uncomfortable feeling in her chest in relation to unhappiness in her work. She was diagnosed with pharyngeal neurosis and given medication, but it did not change her condition. Her menstruation was scanty, and dark in colour.

【Examination】

Pale tongue, thready rapid pulse

【Diagnosis】

Plum pit qi (due to qi stagnation, phlegm retention)

【Treatment Principles】

Regulate the liver, transform phlegm

【Treatment】

RN 22 (*tiān tū*)	RN 17 (*dàn zhōng*)	LV 3 (*tài chōng*)
LI 4 (*hé gǔ*)	ST 36 (*zú sān lǐ*)	PC 6 (*nèi guān*)
ST 40 (*fēng lóng*)	LU 7 (*liè quē*)	

ST 40 (*fēng lóng*) was reduced. Other points were all treated with an even method. Five acupuncture treatments greatly reduced her symptoms.

【Note】

Plum pit qi, mostly seen in women, is a subjective sensation as if a plum pit is stuck in the throat or the throat is compressed, this is usually due to emotional factors. This patient is a good example of this syndrome. Her emotions and feelings of depression cause the liver qi to stagnate, this creates phlegm, which rises upward into the throat. Regulating liver qi and transforming phlegm are the principles for treatment.

LV 3 (*tài chōng*), *yuán*-source of the liver channel, relates to yin, it controls the blood, and can regulate liver qi; LI 4 (*hé gǔ*), *yuán*-source of the large intestine channel, it relates to yang and controls the ascent and descent of qi, thus treating depression. They are commonly called the four-gates and are used to both harmonize qi and blood as well as regulate yin and yang.

RN 17 (*dàn zhōng*), the influential point of qi, circulates the qi of the entire body, together with RN 22 (*tiān tū*) they are used to circulate stagnated qi. "First strengthen the spleen, to prevent it from being involved when the liver is diseased" is the idea behind treating ST 36 (*zú sān lǐ*), *hé*-sea of stomach. This point is selected to strengthen the spleen and stomach in a preventative fashion. ST 40 (*fēng lóng*) strengthens the spleen to aid in the transformation of phlegm.

Geng, female, 17, first visit was on July 14, 1980

【Chief Complaint】

Psycho-emotive issues for 2 weeks

【Present Medical History】

This patient was nervous about her upcoming exams that would allow her to attend college. She was frantically studying and started to become mentally unhinged, about this time she also got her period. She would have moments of clarity, but at other times her thinking was quite disordered. She was restless and easily startled. Taking diazepam and herbal medicine was not effective. She had no desire for food. Her stools were normal.

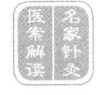

【Examination】

Red tongue with a thick yellowish coating, and a wiry, rapid pulse

【Diagnosis】

Hysteria (due to accumulation of phlegm with heat)

【Treatment Principles】

Regulate qi, remove depression, transform phlegm, open the orifices

【Treatment】

DU 20 (*bǎi huì*)	*sì shén cōng* (EX-HN1)	DU 26 (*rén zhōng*)
RN 17 (*dàn zhōng*)	PC 6 (*nèi guān*)	HT 7 (*shén mén*)
PC 7 (*dà líng*)	SP 6 (*sān yīn jiāo*)	LV 3 (*tài chōng*)

Herbal treatment: Peaceful Palace Bovine Bezoar Pill (*Ān Gōng Niú Huáng Wán* 安宫牛黄丸), one pill each day.

On her 2nd visit, ST 40 (*fēng lóng*) and BL 2 (*cuán zhú*) were added. On her 7th visit, her condition had improved, so DU 26 (*rén zhōng*) was omitted and SI 3 (*hòu xī*) was added. On her 13th visit, DU 20 (*bǎi huì*), *sì shén cōng* (EX-HN1), RN 17 (*dàn zhōng*), PC 6 (*nèi guān*), HT 7 (*shén mén*), SP 6 (*sān yīn jiāo*), and LV 3 (*tài chōng*) were used. After another three treatments she basically recovered.

【Note】

This patient's psycho-emotive problems were due to over thinking and depression. This causes a failure of the liver qi to circulate properly; the spleen also fails in its function of transport and transformation, thus retained fluid turns into phlegm, which disturbs the brain and the mind. This pathology involves the hand *shaoyin* heart, foot *jueyin* liver, and the foot *taiyin* spleen channels. Points from multiple channels should be selected to regulate yin and yang:

DU 20 (*bǎi huì*), *sì shén cōng* (EX-HN1) and DU 26 (*rén zhōng*) are used to open the orifices and wake the spleen. RN 17 (*dàn zhōng*), PC 6 (*nèi guān*), PC 7 (*dà líng*) and HT 7 (*shén mén*) are used to regulate the qi circulation in the chest to calm the mind. SP 6 (*sān yīn jiāo*) strengthens spleen qi, ST 40 (*fēng lóng*) transforms phlegm, LV 3 (*tài chōng*) calms the liver and SI 3 (*hòu xī*) disperses yang qi, sedates the heart and calms the mind.

Summary

Melancholia is caused by emotional injury and qi stagnation, manifesting as being depressed, restless and irritable, crying, and a feeling of blockage in the throat. The principle for treatment is to regulate the *Shĕn*-mind, circulate qi, calm the liver, and remove constraint.

Main points: DU 26 (*rén zhōng*), PC 6 (*nèi guān*), HT 7 (*shén mén*), LV 3 (*tài chōng*).

IMPOTENCE

Lu Shou-yan's Medical Record

Wang, male, 48, first visit was on August 17, 1965

【Chief Complaint】
Impotence and incontinence

【Present Medical History】
This patient took part in the war of liberation in 1947. For an extended period of time, he slept in cold damp places for a long time. These difficult conditions and the hardship of war lead to pain and soreness in the low back, weakness of the four limbs, white urine that at times contained white clumps, painful urination, headaches, and dizziness. He was treated but not cured. From 1959 onward, he suffered from impotence and incontinence.

【Examination】
Pale tongue, soft pulse

【Diagnosis】
Impotence (due to invasion of cold damp, kidney yang deficiency)

【Treatment Principles】
Dispel cold, warm yang, tonify essence

【Treatment】

①	RN 4 (*guān yuán*)	RN 3 (*zhōng jí*)
②	DU 4 (*mìng mén*)	DU 2 (*yāo shù*)
③	BL 23 (*shèn shù*)	

The 3 groups of points were used in turns. Moxibustion with 7 grain-sized cones was done at each point. After 6 times of moxibustion, his impotence was cured and he became energetic again.

【Note】

This case of impotence is caused by invasion of cold damp, exhaustion of the kidney yang along with coldness and deficiency of the essence.

Professor Lu uses the points RN 4 (*guān yuán*) and RN 3 (*zhōng jí*) which are located in the *dantian*, the place where the male essence is stored. Applying moxibustion here dispels the cold from the essence. Moxibustion at DU 4 (*mìng mén*) tonifies the *mingmen* fire. Moxibustion at DU 2 (*yāo shù*) warms *Yù Fáng* (jade house), which is between BL 30 (*bái huán shù*), a point also named *Yù Fáng Shù*, its qi connects with *Yù Fáng* (jade house). The ancient alchemists say "store essence in the jade house". The Back-*shù* points are rooted in the *taiyang* channel and are related to the *du* vessel. Thus, moxibustion at DU 2 (*yāo shù*) can also warm up *Yù Fáng* (jade house). Moxibustion at these two points functions to dispel cold damp from the *du* vessel. Moxibustion at BL 23 (*shèn shù*) tonifies the kidney yang thus producing genuine yin. Six moxibustion treatments using this method improved the patient's energy level and cured the problem.

Cheng Xin-nong's Medical Record

Tao, male, 55, first visit was on October 15, 1985

【Chief Complaint】

Impotence for half a month.

【Present Medical History】

Half a month ago, the patient and his wife got into a quarrel while having sex. After this he could not get an erection, and his testicles began to shrink and pull into this body. Since then he had been depressed, had had a stuffy feeling in his chest, shortness of breath, dizziness, soreness in low back, dry mouth without desire to drink, poor appetite, and poor sleep getting only 2 to 3 hours sleep each night.

【Examination】

Red tongue tip and borders, pulse is wiry and a little rapid, proximal position is weak

【Diagnosis】

Impotence (due to liver stagnation, kidney deficiency)

【Treatment Principles】

Calm the liver to relieve stagnation, tonify kidney yang

【Treatment】

DU 20 (*bǎi huì*)	RN 4 (*guān yuán*)	PC 6 (*nèi guān*)
SP 6 (*sān yīn jiāo*)	LV 3 (*tài chōng*)	

On his first visit, to ease his psychological distress it was explained to him that his problem was only temporary. On the following day, after his first acupuncture treatment the patient reported he was again able to have sex. The above-mentioned treatment was continued and after four treatments he was cured.

【Note】

Collected Treatises of Zhang Jing-yue - Impotence (Jǐng Yüè Quán Shū: Yáng Wěi, 景岳全书 • 阳痿) says: "Impotence is mostly caused by the decline of the *mingmen* fire, the deficiency of essence and qi, or emotional injuries that damage the production of yang qi." *Miraculous Pivot - Tendons (Líng Shū: Jīng Jīn,* 灵枢 • 经筋) says: "The muscle region of the foot *jueyin*, is diseased … the penis fails to act, when caused by endogenous factors it cannot erect."

This patient's impotence stems from emotional factors, this injures the liver, so the yang qi of the liver and kidney cannot open and diffuse. Helping to relieve this patient's worries and fears will help to achieve an effective result. RN 4 (*guān yuán*) is selected to strengthen the kidney yang. SP 6 (*sān yīn jiāo*) is treated to regulate the three yin channels thereby tonifying the yang. DU 20 (*bǎi huì*) is for lifting yang qi, LV 3 (*tài chōng*) is used to smooth the qi of the *jueyin* channel, and PC 6 (*nèi guān*) is selected to sedate the heart and calm the mind.

Summary

Impotence is generally due to over-indulgence in sexual activities, which weakens the *Mìng Mén* (gate of life) fire and exhausts the kidney essence. It may also be due to worries, which damage the heart and spleen; it can also stem from fear and fright which injuries the kidney; or from damp heat driving downward obstructing the ability to get an erection.

Main points: DU 4 (*mìng mén*), BL 23 (*shèn shù*), RN 4 (*guān yuán*), SP 6 (*sān yīn jiāo*).

BL 23 (*shèn shù*) is used to tonify the kidney. DU 4 (*mìng mén*) and RN 4 (*guān yuán*) to replenish the genuine fire of the lower *jiao*. SP 6 (*sān yīn jiāo*) is the intersecting point of the three foot yin channels, which all flow to the lower abdomen and knot together at the external genitals, this point tonifies all the three yin organs.

Add BL 15 (*xīn shù*), HT 7 (*shén mén*), and ST 36 (*zú sān lǐ*) for qi deficiency of the heart and spleen, add LV 2 (*xíng jiān*) and LV 3 (*tài chōng*) for depression, and SP 9 (*yīn líng quán*) can be needled for damp heat driving downward.

HERNIA

Record in *Acupuncture - Moxibustion for Difficult Diseases* (*Qí Nán Zá Bìng Zhēn Jiǔ Zhì Liáo*)

Gao, male, 51, first visit was on June 3, 1994

【Chief Complaint】

Paroxysmal abdominal pain for two days

【Present Medical History】

Two days ago, the patient began to have a paroxysmal abdominal pain with swelling and pain on the left side of the scrotum accompanied by vomiting. No bowel movements for two days.

【Examination】

His abdomen was soft, but slightly bulged and the form of the intestines could be seen. No tenderness or rebound tenderness was present, but there was borborygmus. His tongue was red with a thin coating, pulse was wiry and rapid.

【Diagnosis】

Hernia

【Treatment】

SP 1 (*yǐn bái*)	LV 1 (*dà dūn*)

Moxibustion was applied for 40 minutes each time after needling SP 1 (*yǐn bái*), treatment was given once a day.

With moxibustion, he felt a burning pain in the local area. After seven treatments his swelling and pain disappeared. There was no recurrence.

【Note】

Arcane Essentials from the Imperial Library (*Wài Tái Mì Yào*, 外台秘要) says: "For hernia of the scrotum…, do moxibustion at the medial side of great toe, at the junction of red and white muscle (SP 1) …" *Miraculous Pivot - Channels* says: "foot *jueyin* …, when its qi reverses upward, the testicles are diseased with a hernia; in excess, the hernia is stiff, in deficiency, it is itching. Treat using LV 1 (*dà dūn*)." Following the principle given by the Classics, LV 1 (*dà dūn*) and SP 1 (*yǐn bái*) are selected, and moxibustion is applied to enhance the effect. When the qi of the liver and spleen channels freely circulates, the pain stops as the obstruction has been removed.

Cheng Xin-nong's Medical Record

Li, male, 50, first visit was on January 27, 1992

【Chief Complaint】

Testicle pain for nearly 40 years, aggravated in the past month

【Present Medical History】

The patient reports the pain began when he played football as a young man. His testicles were swollen and painful and were especially worse when tired or attacked by wind. He could not sleep well due to the pain.

【Examination】

Tongue tip was red, coating white, pulse wiry and slippery

【Diagnosis】

Hernia (due to cold damp retention)

【Treatment Principles】

Calm the liver and regulate qi, warm and transform cold damp

【Treatment】

DU 20 (bǎi huì)	RN 4 (guān yuán)	ST 29 (guī lái)
LV 8 (qū quán)	LV 4 (zhōng fēng)	LV 3 (tài chōng)
LV 1 (dà dūn)	SP 6 (sān yīn jiāo)	BL 18 (gān shù)

BL 23 (shèn shù)

Moxibustion was applied to RN 4 (guān yuán). BL 18 (gān shù) and BL 23 (shèn shù) were treated without retaining the needles. Other points were needled with an even method.

With five courses of treatment, the swelling disappeared, only occasional mild pain appeared from time to time. He was basically cured.

【Note】

From his pulse and symptoms, he was seen to have an accumulation of yin qi in the interior and cold damp invasion. His *ren* and liver channels were blocked, leading to the testicles' swelling and pain.

Summary

Hernia is a disease characterized by protrusion of the contents from body cavity, manifesting as swelling and pain of the testicles and scrotum. The causative factors are said to be the invasion of cold, or damp-heat, leading to obstruction of qi and blood in the *ren* and liver channels. Although there are different types of hernia, pain in the lower abdomen is a commonly manifested symptom. The points used to treat come mainly from the *ren* and liver channels. Moxibustion with ginger or direct moxibustion is applied for its treatment.

Main points: RN 4 (*guān yuán*), LV 1 (*dà dūn*), SP 6 (*sān yīn jiāo*).

PROLAPSE OF RECTUM

Shao Jing-ming's Medical Record

Zhao, female, 56, first visit was on August 18, 1977

【Chief Complaint】

Prolapse of rectum for three years

【Present Medical History】

At the beginning, the patient only felt a bearing-down in the anus after bowel movements, after standing up the rectum went back to normal. With the development of disease, the rectum was in a continually prolapsed condition of more than 4 cm. Even coughing or walking would exacerbate the condition. Frequency of bowel movements was increased.

【Examination】

Sallow complexion and listlessness. Pale tongue with white coating, soft weak pulse

【Diagnosis】

Prolapse of rectum (due to sinking of qi of middle *jiao*)

【Treatment Principles】

Lift and reinforce yang qi

【Treatment】

DU 20 (*bǎi huì*)	DU 1 (*cháng qiáng*)	*huán gāng* (EX-CA3)

Acupuncture and moxibustion were applied to DU 20 (*bǎi huì*). The patient should be in a lateral recumbent position when DU 1 (*cháng qiáng*) and *huán gāng* (EX-CA3) are needled. A 3 inch filiform needle was used and inserted to a depth of 2.5 inches. The needle was retained for 20 to 30 minutes, during which time it was manipulated twice to strengthen the needling sensation; this caused the patient to feel a contraction in the anus.

After the first moxibustion treatment, he did not have prolapse when he had a bowel movement. Only a bearing-down sensation appeared when walking, or if he felt tired. One week later, the same moxibustion treatment was given again and the bearing-down sensation disappeared. Another treatment applied to consolidate the effect.

【Note】

This patient has weakness of the spleen and stomach; weakness of the middle *jiao* causes the qi to sink instead of rise, thus the anal prolapse.

Acupuncture and moxibustion at DU 20 (*bǎi huì*) promote yang qi to lift the rectum. DU 1 (*cháng qiáng*) and *huán gāng* (EX-CA3) are the local points near the anus, deep insertion of the needles at this point can strengthen the muscle tone of the anus, regulate the *du* vessel and lift the qi of middle *jiao*.

> *Huán gāng* (EX-CA3) *is located near the anus, at 3 o'clock and 9 o'clock. It is an empirical point for prolapse of the rectum.*

Xiao Shao-qing's Medical Record

Zhu, male, 12, first visit was on May 12, 1956

【Chief Complaint】

Prolapse of the rectum for three years

【Present Medical History】

This patient first experienced prolapse of the rectum three years ago, he had been suffering from chronic enteritis. After treatment the diarrhea was mostly cured, but the prolapse was unchanged. There were accompanying symptoms of dizziness and poor appetite.

【Examination】

Sallow complexion, emaciation, thin white tongue coating, thready weak pulse

【Diagnosis】

Prolapse of the rectum (due to sinking of the qi of the middle *jiao*)

【Treatment Principles】

Tonify qi of the middle *jiao*, lift qi to raise the rectum

【Treatment】

DU 20 (*bǎi huì*)	DU 1 (*cháng qiáng*)	RN 6 (*qì hǎi*)
ST 25 (*tiān shū*)	BL 25 (*dà cháng shù*)	

The tonifying-draining method achieved by rapid insertion and slow withdrawal of the needle was used; needles were retained for 20 minutes. After needling, moxibustion was applied. Treatment was once every other day.

After two treatments, the anus had already contracted, but prolapsed again when passing stools. After six treatments the prolapse was healed, even with carrying heavy loads there was no prolapse. Three more treatments were given to consolidate.

【Note】

The patient has a weak constitution owing to the chronic diarrhea. Sinking of the middle *jiao* qi results in failure of the anus to contract thus resulting in prolapse.

RN 6 (*qì hǎi*) and RN 4 (*guān yuán*) are selected to tonify the qi of the middle *jiao*. Moxibustion at DU 20 (*bǎi huì*) functions to activate the yang qi which lifts the prolapsed rectum. DU 1 (*cháng qiáng*) is needled to strengthen contracture in the anus. ST 25 (*tiān shū*) combined with BL 25 (*dà cháng shù*) regulate the qi of the large intestine thus promoting its normal function.

Summary

Prolapse of the rectum is mostly caused by prolonged diarrhea or dysentery owing to the sinking of the qi of the middle *jiao*. In mild cases, the rectum returns to normal after a bowel movement; in severe cases, coughing or carrying a heavy load will aggravate the prolapse.

Main points: DU 20 (*bǎi huì*), DU 1 (*cháng qiáng*).

RN 6 (*qì hǎi*), ST 36 (*zú sān lǐ*), BL 20 (*pí shù*) and BL 23 (*shèn shù*) are added for those with a weak constitution; moxibustion is applied for cases of yang deficiency.

GYNECOLOGICAL AND PEDIATRIC DISEASES

Internal Diseases

Gynecological and Pediatric Diseases

Diseases of Eyes, Ears, Nose and Throat

Skin Diseases, External Diseases

Others

DYSMENORRHEA

Shao Jing-ming's Medical Record

Li, female, 22

【Chief Complaint】

Dysmenorrhea for eight years

【Present Medical History】

This patient's first menarche was at the age of 14; it was painful. She did not have treatment because the pain was not serious at that time. Four years ago, after being caught in the rain during her period the pain became worse. She took western medicine which stopped the pain, but when menstruating she would still have severe abdominal pain. Her lower abdomen felt cold; she had scanty menstrual flow that was dark in colour with clots. Recently, her menstrual pain was unendurable. Her limbs were cold and there was a cold pain in her lower abdomen. So, she came in for treatment.

【Examination】

Slim build, with a pained expression on her face, sweating from the head; the tongue was slightly dark, with a thin coating, the pulse was wiry

【Diagnosis】

Dysmenorrhea (due to cold stagnated in the uterus)

【Treatment Principles】

Warm the channels to dispel cold, move the qi to activate blood

【Treatment】

RN 4 (*guān yuán*)	SP 6 (*sān yīn jiāo*)	BL 32 (*cì liáo*)

The lifting, thrusting and rotating method of tonification and draining was used. Moxibustion was applied as well.

RN 4 (*guān yuán*) was inserted to a depth of 1.5 inches, causing the arrival of the needle sensation in the perineum. SP 6 (*sān yīn jiāo*) was inserted perpendicularly 1~1.5 inches, causing the needling sensation to travel to the sole of the foot. BL 32 (*cì liáo*) was inserted 1.5~2 inches into the posterior sacral foramen, resulting in the needling sensation to travel to the lower abdomen and perineum.

Her pain was immediately relieved after the arrival of qi and disappeared 10 minutes later. The needle was retained for 30 minutes and manipulated twice in that time. Later, she was treated regularly from 3 to 5 days before her menses till it started, in succession for three periods, after which she was cured. A two year follow-up failed to find any recurrence of the pain.

【Note】

TCM holds that dysmenorrhea is caused by the obstruction of qi and blood. The pathogenic factors leading to obstruction of qi and blood are cold damp retention, liver qi stagnation, qi and blood deficiency and so on. This patient's dysmenorrhea is due to cold obstructed in the uterus. RN 4 (*guān yuán*) is used to tonify the kidney yang to dispel cold, circulate qi and regulate her menstruation. SP 6 (*sān yīn jiāo*) is used to strengthen the spleen to circulate qi and activate blood. BL 32 (*cì liáo*) is to regulate the lower *jiao* and adjust the *chong* and *ren* vessels.

Liang Ci-ming's Medical Record

Yao, female, 23

【Chief Complaint】

Lower abdominal pain during menstruation

【Present Medical History】

Her periods were accompanied by unendurable pain that forced her lay in a fetal position with her knees curled up, and hands pressing on her lower abdomen in order to feel some kind of relief.

【Examination】

Pulse was deep and slow

【Diagnosis】

Dysmenorrhea (due to cold retention, qi stagnation)

【Treatment Principles】

Reinforce qi, invigorate the blood, dispel cold, stop pain

【Treatment】

| Right: | LI 4 (*hé gǔ*) | Left: | SP 6 (*sān yīn jiāo*) |

Even method. The needles were retained for 15 minutes. Treatment caused the pain to stop. Five days later, a follow-up failed to find any recurrence.

【Note】

Pathogenic cold and qi stagnation block the uterus, causing the menstrual flow not to be smooth, thus there is dysmenorrhea. LI 4 (*hé gǔ*) is the *yuán*-source point of the hand *yangming*; it is full of qi and blood. SP 6 (*sān yīn jiāo*) is the point of the foot *taiyin* that is closely related with blood. As the left side is that of blood while the right side is of qi; right LI 4 (*hé gǔ*) and left SP 6 (*sān yīn jiāo*) are used to tonify qi and invigorate blood. When the cold is dispelled, the pain will naturally stop on its own.

Summary

Dysmenorrhea refers to pain in the lower abdomen and low back before, after or during menstruation. Acupuncture - moxibustion is effective for its treatment, not only to immediately stop the pain, but also to improve the long-term condition of the patient. Pain before or during the menstruation is mostly due to the excess syndromes of cold retention and/or qi stagnation; while the pain after menstrual flow is usually from deficiency. Cold excess should be treated by warming the channels to dispel cold; qi stagnation should be treated by regulating qi to remove stasis. Deficiency syndromes should be treated through regulating and tonifying the liver and kidney and by nourishing qi and blood. Acupuncture - moxibustion should be applied once a day, 3 to 5 days before the onset of menstruation, until the flow comes. For those with severe or prolonged cases, acupuncture - moxibustion should be given for at least 3 to 4 cycles.

Main points: RN 4 (*guān yuán*), SP 6 (*sān yīn jiāo*), LV 3 (*tài chōng*).

RN 3 (*zhōng jí*), BL 32 (*cì liáo*) and SP 8 (*dì jī*) are added for those cases of abdominal pain made worse by pressure. PC 6 (*nèi guān*), GB 34 (*yáng líng quán*) and RN 6 (*qì hǎi*) are added for cases of pain which involve the hypochondrium and breasts. BL 23 (*shèn shù*) and ST 36 (*zú sān lǐ*) are added for cases of abdominal pain with soreness in the lower back.

AMENORRHEA

Record in *Acupuncture - Moxibustion for Difficult Diseases* (*Qí Nán Zá Bìng Zhēn Jiǔ Zhì Liáo*)

Yan, female, 43, first visit was on October 12, 1980

【Chief Complaint】
Amenorrhea for half a year

【Present Medical History】
This patient usually has normal menstrual cycles; colour, quantity and quality of the blood are normal. Half a year ago, while she had her cycle she went swimming, and the period suddenly stopped. She had accompanying soreness of the low back, feeling of limb weakness, aversion to wind, headache, and a cold sensation in the lower abdomen. Vaginal discharge was without smell.

【Examination】
Pale tongue with a thin white coating, deep and slow pulse

【Diagnosis】

Amenorrhea (due to cold retention, blood stasis)

【Treatment Principles】

Warm the channels to dispel cold

【Treatment】

Point:	RN 4 (*guān yuán*)		
Herbs:	胡椒	*hú jiāo*	Fructus Piperis
	丁香	*dīng xiāng*	Flos Caryophylli
	肉桂	*Ròu guì*	Cortex Cinnamomi

Moxibustion was applied at RN 4 (*guān yuán*) using a "cake" made of the above herbs. Six cones of moxa were burned. On the following day, she said her menstruation started again.

【Note】

Synopsis of Prescriptions of the Golden Chamber - Women's Miscellaneous Diseases (Jīn Guì Yào Luè: Fù Rén Zá Bìng, 金匮要略 • 妇人杂病) says: "Women's diseases are due to deficiency, accumulation of cold, and stagnation of qi; menstruation stops." RN 4 (*guān yuán*) is the intersecting point of the *ren* vessel and the three foot yin channels, additionally it is the place from where the qi of the *san jiao* originates; it is one of those points that can tonify the whole body. The herbs *hú jiāo* (*Fructus Piperis*), *dīng xiāng* (*Flos Caryophylli*) and *ròu guì* (*Cortex Cinnamomi*) are pungent and warm medicinals, they warm the channels and dispel cold to stop pain. They strengthen kidney yang, dispel cold, unobstruct the channels and regulate the *ren* to smooth the menstrual flow.

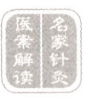

Cheng Xin-nong's Medical Record

Hu, female, 40, first visit was on January 3, 1992

【Chief Complaint】

Amenorrhea for two years

【Present Medical History】

Two years ago, the patient had a quarrel with someone during her menses; prior to this she had been depressed and her periods were becoming increasingly irregular. There were accompanying symptoms of lower abdominal distention, cold pain in the loins that radiated to the back, fullness in chest, sighing, irritability, limbs numbness and loose stools 2 to 3 times a day.

【Examination】

Patient's cheeks and lips were dark purple; tongue was purplish with a thin yellow coating, and pulse wiry, proximal position was weak.

【Diagnosis】

Amenorrhea (due to qi stagnation with blood stasis)

【Treatment Principles】

Regulate the qi, remove stasis

【Treatment】

RN 17 (*dàn zhōng*)	RN 6 (*qì hǎi*)	RN 3 (*zhōng jí*)
LI 4 (*hé gǔ*)	SP 10 (*xuè hǎi*)	SP 6 (*sān yīn jiāo*)
LV 3 (*tài chōng*)	LV 2 (*xíng jiān*)	

RN 3 (*zhōng jí*) was treated with moxibustion, other points were needled with an even method.

She insisted on seven courses of treatment, although these were not on a regular timescale. Her menstruation started again with regular cycles; the other symptoms disappeared.

【Note】

Concerning emotional factors, anger damages the liver causing qi stagnation that leads to blood stasis; so the menstruation stops. The free flow of qi and blood is blocked, so she has pain in her back, loins and numbness of the limbs. Prolonged stagnation produces heat, so she has irritability and a yellow tongue coating.

Summary

Amenorrhea, if due to exhaustion of the blood which can be caused by bleeding, over-indulgence in sexual activities, multiple childbirth or prolonged disease, is known as exhaustive amenorrhea; if due to emotional causes like anger or invasion of cold, is known as stasis amenorrhea.

Main points: RN 4 (*guān yuán*), SP 6 (*sān yīn jiāo*), SP 10 (*xuè hǎi*).

BL 20 (*pí shù*), BL 23 (*shèn shù*), RN 6 (*qì hǎi*) and ST 36 (*zú sān lǐ*) are added for exhaustive amenorrhea to tonify kidney qi, strengthen the spleen and stomach and replenish yin and blood.

RN 3 (*zhōng jí*), LI 4 (*hé gǔ*) and LV 2 (*xíng jiān*) are added for stasis amenorrhea to reduce heat and remove stasis to produce new blood. Moxibustion is used for the cases with cold.

Bēng Lòu (UTERINE BLEEDING)

Cheng Xin-nong's Medical Record

Liu, female, 31, first visit was on May 13, 1992

【Chief Complaint】
Prolonged menstruation for 14 days

【Present Medical History】
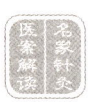
Fourteen days ago, this patient's menstrual flow began, it was light in colour and accompanied by soreness in the lumbar region. She took some Chinese medicine but it was not effective. She had her first period at the age of 14. The cycle, colour and quantity of her menstruation were all normal. She got married at the age of 27, and has had two abortions within her two

years of marriage. She was always tired, afraid of cold, mentally fatigued and does not like to talk.

【Examination】

Pale complexion, pale tongue with a thin coating, and a deep thready pulse

【Diagnosis】

Uterine bleeding (*Bēng Lòu*) (due to deficiency of *chong* and *ren* vessels, kidney qi deficiency)

【Treatment Principles】

Regulate and tonify the *chong* and *ren* vessels, tonify qi to control blood

【Treatment】

DU 20 (*bǎi huì*)	RN 4 (*guān yuán*)	ST 36 (*zú sān lǐ*)
SP 6 (*sān yīn jiāo*)	SJ 4 (*yáng chí*)	SP 1 (*yǐn bái*)

SP 1 (*yǐn bái*) was treated with moxibustion; other points were needled using a tonifying method.

After five treatments, the uterine bleeding was reduced and she felt better emotionally and physical strength was better. After seven treatments, the bleeding stopped. Another seven treatments consolidated her condition and all her symptoms disappeared.

【Note】

The two abortions damaged her *chong* and *ren* vessels. Not taking care of one's health causes qi and blood deficiency, thus the weakness of the *chong* and *ren* vessels, the liver and spleen lose their controlling and storing functions, hence the uterine bleeding.

DU 20 (*bǎi huì*) is used to lift the qi of the middle *jiao*. RN 4 (*guān yuán*) is used to tonify the *yuán*-source qi to regulate the *chong* and *ren* vessels; ST 36 (*zú sān lǐ*), SP 6 (*sān yīn jiāo*), SP 1 (*yǐn bái*) are used to harmonize liver and spleen to restore their functions in controlling and storing blood and replenish qi and blood; SJ 4 (*yáng chí*) is the *yuán*-source point of *sanjiao* channel, functioning to regulate the *penetrating* and *ren* vessels and reinforce qi to control blood.

Xiao Shao-qing's Medical Record

Huang, female, 24, first visit was on May 19, 1998

【Chief Complaint】

Irregular menstruation accompanied by *Bēng Lòu* (uterine bleeding) for seven years

【Present Medical History】

This patient was 15 at menarche. The cycle, colour and quantity of her menstruation were all normal. Since 1992, the cycle became disordered, she would have it once every two or three months, even up to six months between periods. The flow was profuse, even after she had bled for seven days and contained big clots. Hundreds of doses of herbal medicine, hormone therapy, and three D&C's failed to have any effect. Presently she had irregular cycles that lasted for more than seven days with scanty dark flow, distending pain in lower abdomen, large clots, accompanied by dizziness, headache, and palpitations.

【Examination】

Sallow complexion, yellow and slight greasy tongue coating, thready and rapid pulse

【Diagnosis】

Uterine bleeding (*Bēng Lòu*) (due to liver qi stagnation, failure of the spleen in transportation and transformation)

【Treatment Principles】

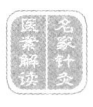

Calm the liver and regulate qi, strengthen the spleen and replenish blood, regulate the *chong* and *ren* vessels

【Treatment】

Acupuncture, moxibustion and herbal medicine were used in combination.

Points:

① DU 20 (*bǎi huì*)	PC 6 (*nèi guān*)	RN 12 (*zhōng wǎn*)
ST 25 (*tiān shū*)	RN 6 (*qì hǎi*)	RN 4 (*guān yuán*)
ST 30 (*qì chōng*)	SP 10 (*xuè hǎi*)	SP 8 (*dì jī*)
SP 6 (*sān yīn jiāo*)	LV 3 (*tài chōng*)	
② DU 23 (*shàng xīng*)	LI 4 (*hé gǔ*)	RN 8 (*shén què*)
RN 4 (*guān yuán*)	ST 36 (*zú sān lǐ*)	SP 4 (*gōng sūn*)
SP 1 (*yǐn bái*)	KI 3 (*tài xī*)	ST 28 (*shuǐ dào*)
ST 29 (*guī lái*)	LV 14 (*qī mén*)	

RN 6 (*qì hǎi*) was needled through to RN 4 (*guān yuán*).

The two groups of points were alternately used in turn. They were needled using an even method and retained for 30 minutes. During this time the Phoenix Flying technique was used to stimulate the needles once every 10 minutes. At the same time, RN 12 (*zhōng wǎn*), RN 8 (*shén què*), ST 25 (*tiān shū*), RN 6 (*qì hǎi*) and RN 4 (*guān yuán*) were treated with cupping for 5 to 10 minutes. Treatment was given once a day, one month being one course of treatment.

Medicines:

① *Dān Zhī Xiāo Yáo Wán*	Augmented Free and Easy Wanderer Pill 丹栀逍遥丸	
② *Guī Pí Wán*	Restore the Spleen Pill 归脾丸	

The two medicines were taken together, twice a day, 4g each time, to strengthen the spleen and control blood.

Seven courses of treatment, 210 treatments in all together, brought her cycle into some semblance of regularity with about 40 days between periods; the quantity, colour and quality of the flow were all improved.

It lasted five to eight days, medium quantity, fresh red colour, small dark clots, and without being prolonged.

【Note】

This patient suffered from irregular menstruation accompanied by *Bēng Lòu* for seven years. She is introverted and was depressed for a long time, this caused the liver to become disordered, resulting in a qi stagnation and inability of the *chong* and *ren* to store blood. Because of the liver's disorder, her menstruation was delayed. *Restoration of Health from the Myriad Diseases* (*Wàn Bìng Huí Chūn*, 万病回春) says: "Menstruation that comes late, dark and with clots, due to qi stagnation and blood stasis." The Treatment principles are to calm the liver, regulate qi and invigorate the blood to regulate menstruation. *Treatment of Diseases in Verse* says: "For menstruation not in regular cycles, SP 8 (*dì jī*) and SP 10 (*xuè hǎi*) are the points to treat." SP 8 (*dì jī*) is the *xī*-cleft point of the foot *taiyin* spleen channel; used together with SP 10 (*xuè hǎi*) they invigorate the blood, regulate menstruation, and circulate qi to stop pain. LV 14 (*qī mén*), LV 3 (*tài chōng*), ST 28 (*shuǐ dào*), and ST 29 (*guī lái*) are drained to calm the liver, regulate qi, and invigorate the blood to smooth the menstrual flow. When the liver is regulated and the stomach harmonized, the menstruation comes regularly. The *chong* vessel is the sea of blood, the *ren* vessel is responsible for nourishing the fetus. Should they be disordered, the sea of blood will not be capable of storing blood, thus the uterine bleeding occurs.

RN 12 (*zhōng wǎn*), RN 8 (*shén què*), RN 6 (*qì hǎi*), RN 4 (*guān yuán*), ST 30 (*qì chōng*), ST 36 (*zú sān lǐ*), SP 6 (*sān yīn jiāo*) and SP 1 (*yǐn bái*) can all be selected for treatment. Acupuncture together with moxibustion functions to regulate the *chong* and *ren* vessels, reinforce the qi of the middle *jiao*, and strengthen the spleen promoting its function of controlling the blood. This patient has had uterine bleeding for a long time; her qi and blood are deficient, the heart and brain lack nourishment, which manifests as dizziness, headache and palpitations. The head is the intersection of all yang channels, the face is the primarily nourished by the *yangming* channels. DU 20 (*bǎi huì*) is used together with the *yuán*-source and *hé*-sea points of the hand *yangming* large intestine channel to tonify and rise the clean yang to

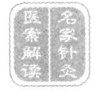

dispel wind and stop pain. PC 6 (*nèi guān*) opens the *yinwei mai*, SP 4 (*gōng sūn*) opens the *chong* vessel, they are tonified to treat palpitations due to the heart/mind being disordered. KI 3 (*tài xī*) is the *yuán*-source point of the foot *shaoyin* kidney channel, it is tonified to nourish kidney yin which in turn subdues deficient fire. DU 23 (*shàng xīng*) is tonified to activate the yang qi of the *du* vessel to assist DU 20 (*bǎi huì*) in dispelling wind and stopping pain. The combination of acupuncture with herbal treatment functions to calm the liver, regulate qi, strengthen the spleen, replenish blood, strengthen the qi of the middle *jiao*, and regulate the *chong* and *ren* vessels. In this way the patient's long term menstrual problem is cured.

Summary

Uterine bleeding (*Bēng Lòu* 崩漏) can be caused by excessive worry, blood stasis, and invasion of either cold or heat, causing a failure of the *chong* and *ren* vessels in their function of consolidating, and the liver and spleen in their functions of storing and controlling blood. The basic treatment principles are to tonify the *chong* and *ren* vessels, regulate the liver and spleen, and augment qi to control blood.

Points: DU 20 (*bǎi huì*), RN 4 (*guān yuán*), BL 18 (*gān shù*), BL 20 (*pí shù*), SP 6 (*sān yīn jiāo*), SP 1 (*yǐn bái*), SJ 4 (yang *chí*).

Add DU 4 (*mìng mén*) and RN 6 (*qì hǎi*) to treat cold syndrome; promote the qi to dispel cold. Add SP 10 (*xuè hǎi*) and KI 5 (*shuǐ quán*) for heat syndrome to clear heat from blood. Add RN 3 (*zhōng jí*) and LV 3 (*tài chōng*) for blood stasis syndrome to remove stasis to produce new blood.

Rǔ Pǐ (BREAST NODULES)

Guo Cheng-jie's Medical Records

Female, 40, first visit was on May 6, 1980

【Chief Complaint】

Breast pain with nodules for six years

【Present Medical History】

Six years ago, this patient had an abortion after which her menstrual cycle became erratic and she started to have breast swelling and pain. By taking Chinese herbal medicine the pain could be relieved, but it would start again when she stopped taking the herbs. In the past three years 15 days before the onset of her menstrual flow, she would feel numbness on the tip of the tongue and stiffness of the tongue root. At night on the 2nd to 3rd days of the menses, she had a salty taste in her in mouth and spit out about 10ml of blood. She was irritable, usually had a hot temper, late onset of her period along with scanty, pale flow and breast pain that was worse before the period and when she was angry or tired. Additionally, she had symptoms of a frontal headache, difficulty in falling asleep, dream-disturbed sleep, blurred vision, tinnitus, pain and weakness of the lower back, distending pain in hypochondria, bitter taste in the mouth, and throat dryness.

【Examination】

She was thin with a pale complexion. Her breasts were normal in appearance, no exudation from nipples. Patchy, movable and smooth masses, 4.5cm × 3.5cm, with medium hardness, clear margins, and significant tenderness, were felt in the laterosuperior parts of her breasts. The cervical and subaxillary lymph nodes were enlarged. Her tongue was red, not moist, with a thin white coating, and a wiry thready pulse.

【Diagnosis】

Breast nodules (*Rǔ Pǐ*) (due to liver kidney yin deficiency)

【Treatment Principles】

Reinforce the liver and kidney, regulate the *chong* and *ren* vessels.

【Treatment】

①	SI 11 (*tiān zōng*)	GB 21 (*jiān jǐng*)	BL 18 (*gān shù*)

BL 23 (*shèn shù*)

②   ST 15 (*wū yì*)   RN 17 (*dàn zhōng*)   SP 6 (*sān yīn jiāo*)

KI 3 (*tài xī*)

The two point groups were alternately treated once a day; 10 treatments constituting one course of treatment with four days of rest before the next course. After five courses of treatment the pain in her breasts before menstruation disappeared, the masses decreased to 0.5 cm × 0.5 cm, and the tenderness disappeared. She no longer had the abnormal taste in her mouth during menstruation, nor irritability and stopped spitting blood. She did, however, still have the dry throat, difficulty in falling asleep, and weakness of the low back. Two more courses of treatment cured all her symptoms. Three years later, the follow-up showed no recurrence.

【Note】

This patient's menstrual issues were differentiated as a deficiency of the liver and kidney yin and disharmony of the *chong* and *ren* vessels. ST 15 (*wū yì*) and RN 17 (*dàn zhōng*) were selected to regulate the channels that run through the breast and to invigorate the blood. BL 18 (*gān shù*) is used to directly smooth the liver qi and, add GB 21 (*jiān jǐng*), because of its interior/exterior relationship to the liver, to regulate the gallbladder qi in order to smooth the liver qi. SI 11 (*tiān zōng*) is effective in removing obstructions from the channels and collaterals, and is good for treating breast diseases. BL 23 (*shèn shù*) and KI 3 (*tài xī*) nourish kidney water and supplement kidney yin. SP 6 (*sān yīn jiāo*) is selected to strengthen the spleen and stomach, tonify the liver and kidney, regulate qi and blood, and remove obstructions from the channels and collaterals. This combination of points functions to subdue swelling, transform masses and stop pain.

Female, 25, first visit was on March 17, 1999

【Chief Complaint】

Distending pain in breasts for eight months

【Present Medical History】

Eight months ago, after getting angry with someone, she began to have a distending pain in the breasts. Afterwards the pain repeatedly appeared and got worse before menstruation. Masses were felt in the breasts. Recently, she had delayed menstruation which was accompanied by distending pain in the abdomen.

【Examination】

A patch-like 3.5 cm × 3.5 cm mass was felt in the laterosuperior part of the right breast, and a 2.5 cm × 2.5 cm mass was felt in the laterosuperior part of the left breast. They were movable, smooth and tender. The subaxillary lymphnodes were not examined. She had a pale red tongue, and wiry pulse. Infrared scanning showed hyperplasia of the mammary glands.

【Diagnosis】

Breast nodules (*Rŭ Pĭ*) (due to liver qi stagnation)

【Treatment Principles】

Calm the liver, regulate qi, soften and transform masses

【Treatment】

ST 15 (*wū yì*)	ST 18 (*rŭ gēn*)	LI 4 (*hé gŭ*)

GB 34 (*yáng líng quán*)

Electric stimulation was applied for 30 minutes. After the first treatment, she felt much relieved and it put her in a good mood. After three treatments the masses became much smaller and softer. Six treatments cured her completely.

【Note】

This was a case of liver qi stagnation.

Female, 42, first visit was on March 30, 1999

【Chief Complaint】

A dull pain and masses in the breasts for one month

【Present Medical History】

She had a ten-year history of hyperplasia of the mammary glands that was controlled by acupuncture - moxibustion and herbal treatment. Recently, the pain started again after she felt fatigued. Now her entire body felt tired, accompanied by soreness and weakness in low back and knees, dizziness, blurred vision, and poor appetite.

【Examination】

Sallow complexion, patch-like, movable and smooth masses, 5 cm × 4 cm, with clear margins, tenderness; felt in the laterosuperior parts of breasts. The cervical and subaxillary lymph nodes were not examined. This patient had a pale tongue; deep thready pulse.

【Diagnosis】

Breast nodules (*Rǔ Pǐ*) (due to qi and blood deficiency)

【Treatment Principles】

Replenish qi and blood, circulate qi and invigorate the blood

【Treatment】

①	ST 15 (*wū yì*)	ST 18 (*rǔ gēn*)	ST 36 (*zú sān lǐ*)
②	GB 21 (*jiān jǐng*)	SI 11 (*tiān zōng*)	BL 20 (*pí shù*)

ST 36 (*zú sān lǐ*) and BL 20 (*pí shù*) were tonified, other points were treated with an even method. The needles were retained for 30 minutes. Two groups of points were alternately used, treatment was given once a day. A modified verision of *Shèng Yù Tāng* (Sage Healing Decoction, 圣愈汤) was prescribed.

After five treatments, the pain was relieved and the masses began to soften and shrink, however the symptoms of qi deficiency still existed. The same treatment procedure was continued for another seven treatments, after which the pain and masses disappeared. Because she lived far from the clinic, she discontinued the acupuncture treatments, but did take 10 packets of herb medicine home. The follow-up next month showed no re-occurrence.

【Note】

This was a syndrome of qi and blood deficiency.

Young girl, 12, first visit was on June 10, 1980

【Chief Complaint】

Pain and breast masses for three months

【Present Medical History】

This patient had extreme breast tenderness. She could not even stand for her breasts to touch her desk when studying at school. Pain killers were ineffective.

【Examination】

This patient's development was normal; the complexion a little sallow, but with luster. The colour of the breasts was normal, but there were hard, movable nodules with clear margins, 2 cm in size below the nipples, along with significant tenderness. Tongue slightly red, pulse normal.

【Diagnosis】

Normal adolescent development of a young girl

【Treatment Principles】

Circulate qi, invigorate the blood, disperse masses, stop pain

【Treatment】

RN 17 (*dàn zhōng*)	ST 15 (*wū yì*)	LI 4 (*hé gǔ*)

An even method was applied. Needles retained for 15 minutes. Treatment was giving once every other day. After six treatments, she reported the pain had eased to a considerable degree and the masses had become softer. Four treatments cured her completely. Six months later, the follow-up found no recurrence.

【Note】

This is a young woman's *Rǔ Pǐ* (mammary development problem)

Male, 57, first visit was on January 8, 1999

【Chief Complaint】

Left breast pain, with a mass in it for five months

【Present Medical History】

At the beginning, he just felt pain in his left breast that gradually got worse; taking anodyne was no use. One month later, the left breast began to be enlarged and there was a palpable mass. He was generally in a hot temper.

【Examination】

The left breast was obvious enlarged, its nipple and colour were normal, a flat mass, 2 cm × 0.8 cm in size, was felt under the mammary areola. The mass was medium hard movable, smooth, and with obvious tenderness. The cervical and subaxillary lymph nodes were not enlarged. Slightly dark tongue, thin white coating, wiry and a bit slow pulse.

【Diagnosis】

Mammary development problem of males

【Treatment Principles】

Calm the liver and regulate qi, stop pain, disperse masses

【Treatment】

RN 17 (dàn zhōng)	ST 15 (wū yì)	LI 4 (hé gǔ)

BL 18 (gān shù)

Reducing method. After seven acupuncture treatments, the pain stopped and the mass became soft. After 15 treatments the mass was reduced to 0.5 cm×0.5 cm. After two months, the follow-up found no recurrence of pain and the mass disappeared.

【Note】

This is a male *Rǔ Pǐ* (breast nodules). It is due to liver qi stagnation, causing blood stasis, and thus the formation of a mass.

Summary

According to Professor Guo Cheng-jie *Rǔ Pǐ* (乳癖), breast nodules or masses, hyperplasia, or adolescent mammary development problems with pain that is aggravated before menstruation, or by emotional upset or fatigue is due to liver qi stagnation and obstruction of qi in the foot *yangming* stomach channel. The liver functions to maintain the free flow of qi and stores blood, its channel distributes to the chest and connects with the breast. The stomach channel of the foot *yangming* passes through the breast. In cases where worry damages the spleen causing a failure in its ability to transport and transform; or where anger damages the liver, causing liver qi stagnation, which obstructs the qi and blood circulation of liver and stomach, leading to disharmony in the *chong* and *ren* vessels; nodules will be formed in the breasts. The treatment begins with moving qi, treating the liver and stomach, and regulating the *penetrating* and *ren* vessels. Based on the individual conditions of patients in clinic, Professor Guo divides it into the following four syndromes:

a. Liver qi stagnation: distending pain and masses in the breasts that get worse before menstruation or during episodes of anger. Pain radiates to the subaxillary region, shoulder and back, and is accompanied by fullness in the chest, abdominal distention, poor appetite, irregular menstruation, tongue not red, pulse wiry.

b. Liver fire: distending pain with a burning sensation in the breasts and hypochondria made worse by pressure, there is irritability and irascibility, a bitter taste in the mouth, a dry throat, early arrival of menstruation, yellow urination, yellow tongue coating, and a wiry, rapid pulse.

c. Liver and kidney yin deficiency: masses and pain in the breasts, sometimes better and sometimes worse, dizziness, blurred vision, dry mouth, hot sensation in the five centers, red tongue with a sparse coating, thready, wiry and rapid pulse.

d. *Qi* and blood deficiency: nodules in the breasts, dull pain, worse with fatigue, poor appetite, dizziness, blurred vision, palpitations, pale complexion, pale tongue, deep thready pulse.

Main points: on the chest: ST 15 (*wū yì*), RN 17 (*dàn zhōng*), LI 4 (*hé gǔ*); on the back: GB 21 (*jiān jǐng*), SI 11 (*tiān zōng*), BL 18 (*gān shù*).

Add LV 3 (*tài chōng*) for liver fire. For yin deficiency syndrome omit LI 4 (*hé gǔ*), add KI 3 (*tài xī*). For qi and blood deficiency omit LI 4 (*hé gǔ*), add ST 36 (*zú sān lǐ*) and BL 20 (*pí shù*). For irregular menstruation add SP 6 (*sān yīn jiāo*).

These two groups of points were alternately used once a day. Lifting, thrusting and rotating techniques were used to tonify and drain with needles being retained for 20 to 30 minutes. Ten treatments constituted one course with three to four days of rest between courses. No acupuncture was given during menstruation.

ST 15 (*wū yì*) located on the breast and RN 17 (*dàn zhōng*) which is lateral to breast are used to unobstruct channel qi and invigorate the blood of the breast. BL 18 (*gān shù*) circulates liver qi it is assisted by GB 21 (*jiān jǐng*), which due to the exterior/interior relationship of these two organs, circulates gall bladder qi to regulate liver qi. LI 4 (*hé gǔ*) the *yuán*-source of the hand *yangming* and ST 36 (*zú sān lǐ*) the *hé*-sea of the foot *yangming* are used together to conduct the qi of the hand and foot *yangming* channels, nourish stomach and strengthen the spleen, strengthen the post-heaven foundation of the body, enhance resistance to disease and prevent liver fire from affecting the stomach. SI 11 (*tiān zōng*) is effective for breast diseases as it removes obstructions from the channels and collaterals by soothing the liver and regulating the qi in the *yangming*. LV 3 (*tài chōng*) clears liver fire, BL 20 (*pí shù*) strengthens the spleen causing qi and blood to flourish, KI 3 (*tài xī*) replenishs kidney water to supplement liver yin, SP 6 (*sān yīn jiāo*) enhances the spleen and stomach, benefits the liver and kidney, regulates qi and blood, and removes obstructions from the channels and collaterals.

Lòu Rǔ (ABNORMAL LACTATION)

He Pu-ren's Medical Record

Chen, female, 30, visited on May 29, 2002

【Chief Complaint】
Lòu Rǔ (abnormal lactation) for two years

【Present Medical History】
Two years ago, she began to suffer abnormal lactation. Milk would flow out when the breasts were pressed. The breasts were normal in colour, without swelling or pain, nor were there any masses. She had scanty menstruation that was pale in colour and only lasted for two days. In the past two years, she gained nearly 10kg. She went to the Gynecological Department of Peking Union Medical College Hospital for treatment. The

examination showed that her prolactin was normal; infrared scanning showed mild hyperplasia of the mammary glands. An MRI of the head showed everything was normal. She was thought to be suffering from an endocrine dysfunction, so no particular medicine was administered for her.

【Anamnesis】

A history of hypertension for two years

【Examination】

The breasts were normal in appearance without redness, swelling or hard nodules. Pale tongue, white coating, deep thready pulse.

【Diagnosis】

Abnormal lactation (*Lòu Rǔ*) (due to liver stagnation, spleen deficiency)

【Treatment Principles】

Calm the liver, strengthen the spleen, replenish qi and blood, regulate the *chong* and *ren* vessels

【Treatment】

GB 41 (*zú lín qì*)

Acupuncture with one inch filiform needle, which was retained for 30 minutes. Twice a week. After the first treatment, her abnormal lactation was greatly reduced. Five treatments cured her. The follow-up for one year showed no recurrence.

【Note】

Lòu Rǔ refers to an abnormal lactation without infant's sucking. Its pathogenesis is qi and blood deficiency, *yangming* qi non-consolidation, or liver channel blockage due to accumulated heat. Qi stagnation forces milk out of the breasts. This patient has hypertension; long term emotional factors constrained her liver, thus disordering the free flow of qi.

Through the exterior/interior relationship between the liver and gallbladder needling GB 41 (*zú lín qì*) can smooth liver qi. When liver keeps its normal free flow of qi, the milk secretion will be controlled. GB 41 (*zú*

lín qì) is one of the eight confluent points; it opens the *dai*-girdling vessel. Menstruation, pregnancy, delivery, and lactation are all closely related to proper functioning of the *chong*, *ren* and *du* vessels that are tied together and influenced by the *dai* vessel. Therefore GB 41 (*zú lín qì*) is treated to regulate the functions of the *chong*, *ren* and *dai* vessels; strengthening qi and blood to control milk secretion. Professor He uses GB 41 (*zú lín qì*) as a single point to calm the liver, strengthen the spleen, strengthen qi and blood, and treat abnormal lactation (*Lòu Rǔ*) with a remarkable effect. Should there be bloody secretions, the patient should be screened for breast cancer.

Rǔ Nǜ (THELORRHAGIA)

Guo Cheng-jie's Medical Record

Zhang, female, 45, first visit was on March 2, 1982

【Chief Complaint】
Bleeding from the right nipple for three months

【Present Medical History】
The bleeding was gradually worse, and without pain. One month ago, she was diagnosed with a tumor in the mammary duct. Unwilling to have an operation, she came for acupuncture-moxibustion treatment. Her menstrual cycle was irregular and with scanty flow. She was frequently irritable and had insomnia.

【Examination】
This patient felt dejected. The breasts were symmetrical, nipple and areola were normal in colour, profuse pink fluid was leaking out from the right nipple and would squirt out when the breast was pressed. No nodules were found. Dark tongue with a yellowish coating, wiry pulse.

【Diagnosis】

Thelorrhagia (*Rǔ Nǜ*) (due to liver stagnation transformed into fire)

【Treatment Principles】

Calm the liver and regulate qi, strengthen spleen to control blood

【Treatment】

①	ST 15 (*wū yì*)	ST 18 (*rǔ gēn*)	LI 4 (*hé gǔ*)
	ST 36 (*zú sān lǐ*)		
②	BL 18 (*gān shù*)	BL 17 (*gé shù*)	BL 20 (*pí shù*)

BL 17 (*gé shù*), BL 20 (*pí shù*), and ST 36 (*zú sān lǐ*) were tonified; the other points were drained.

The two groups of points were used in turns. Treatment was given once a day.

After 10 acupuncture treatments, although the quantity of discharge from the nipple was not reduced, the colour became lighter. After another 10 treatments the bleeding was reduced and when the breast was pressed, the discharge no longer squirted out. The treatment was continued and the herbal decoction *Dān Zhī Xiāo Yáo Sǎn* (Moutan Bark and Cape Jasmine Fruit Free Wanderer Powder, 丹栀逍遥散) was also prescribed, one dose everyday. In total she had three courses of treatment and eight doses of herbal medicine, after which there was no more bleeding when the breast was pressed. It was cured for the short-term. Three months later, the follow-up found no recurrence.

【Note】

This is a case of mammary cancer. It is differentiated as liver qi stagnation transforming to fire, secondary to emotions constraining the liver qi; the liver overacts on the spleen, which fails to control blood, and the heat forces the blood from the breast.

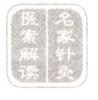

MACROMASTIA

Guo Cheng-jie's Medical Record

Wang, female, 28, first visit was on August 3, 1980

【Chief Complaint】

Breasts quickly enlarged in the past two months

【Present Medical History】

This patient had breast-fed for one year after the birth of her child, after which she was weaned. Before the onset of this problem her menstruation was normal, but half a year after weaning the breasts grew larger than when she was breast feeding. She felt heavy with a bearing-down sensation, but without pain.

【Examination】

She had an average figure. The breasts enlarged to the point where they reached down to the costal margin with the nipples extending down to the middle part of abdomen. The mammary glands were soft, with irregular nodules in them, no tenderness or abnormal colour. The subaxillary lymph nodes were not palpated. She was irritable, had a hot temper, and slept poorly. Pale red tongue, thready and lax pulse.

【Diagnosis】

Macromastia

【Treatment Principles】

Calm the liver, circulate qi, regulate the *chong* and *ren* vessels

【Treatment】

①   ST 15 (*wū yì*)   RN 17 (*dàn zhōng*)   LI 4 (*hé gǔ*)

	SP 6 (*sān yīn jiāo*)		
②	GB 21 (*jiān jǐng*)	SI 11 (*tiān zōng*)	BL 18 (*gān shù*)

An even method. Two groups were used alternately. Treatment was given once a day, with the needles being retained for 30 minutes.

After five treatments the distention and bearing-down sensation was relieved. After one course of treatment, the breasts began to shrink. After 4 courses, the breasts retracted to the lateral border of the chest and the nipples to the 6th rib, returning to the size they were when she was breast-feeding, the glands were rich and soft, and no nodules were felt.

【Note】

Differentiation: this patient's breast enlargement is due to liver qi stagnation. Unsmooth flow of qi and blood in the liver and stomach channels causes blood obstruction, leading to disharmony of the *chong* and *ren* vessels, which results in the leaking of qi and blood and disordered nourishment of the breasts.

Yīn Tǐng (PROLAPSE OF UTERUS)

Record in *Acupuncture - Moxibustion for Difficult Diseases* (*Qí Nán Zá Bìng Zhēn Jiǔ Zhì Liáo*)

Gao, 50, female, first visit was on June 15, 1986

【Chief Complaint】

Prolapse of uterus for many years

【Present Medical History】

A bearing-down sensation in the lower abdomen aggravated by fatigue and standing for a prolonged period of time, listlessness, palpitations, shortness of breath, achy lower back, frequent urination, profuse leucorrhea. Gynecological examination: Prolapse of uterus in degree I.

【Diagnosis】

Prolapse of uterus (*Yīn Tǐng*) (due to qi deficiency, sinking of qi)

【Treatment Principles】

Lift yang to raise prolapse

【Treatment】

DU 20 (*bǎi huì*)	RN 6 (*qì hǎi*)	GB 28 (*wéi dào*)
ST 25 (*tiān shū*)	ST 29 (*guī lái*)	

ST 25 (*tiān shū*) needled through to ST 29 (*guī lái*). Treatment was given once a day, 12 treatments constituting one course. After three courses of treatment, she felt some relief in the bearing-down sensation. After another three courses, the uterus was restored to its normal position.

【Note】

DU 20 (*bǎi huì*), located on the top of the head, can be used to treat lower disease in the lower part of the body and lift prolapse. RN 6 (*qì hǎi*) tonifies qi to restore the prolapsed uterus. GB 28 (*wéi dào*), the intersecting point of the foot *shaoyang* gallbladder with the *dai* vessel, acts to tighten and stabilize the uterus. ST 25 (*tiān shū*) needled through to ST 29 (*guī lái*) strengthens the lower abdominal muscles and helps to hold the uterus in place.

Summary

Yīn Tǐng (阴挺), prolapse of uterus, refers to descent of the uterus into the vagina. Usually it is the result of liver stagnation, with sinking of qi due to spleen deficiency. In most cases symptoms of deficiency are present. But sometimes damp heat flowing into the liver channel is seen, this is accompanied with hesitant urination, and irritability with internal heat.

Main points: DU 20 (*bǎi huì*), GB 28 (*wéi dào*), RN 4 (*guān yuán*), and SP 6 (*sān yīn jiāo*).

Add RN 6 (*qì hǎi*) and ST 36 (*zú sān lǐ*) for qi and blood deficiency.

GB 28 (*wéi dào*) is needled with the tip of the needle pointing toward the uterus. It can be needled to a depth of two to three inches, with a medium or strong stimulation. Treat once everyday or every other day; seven treatments constitutes one course.

ENURESIS

Cheng Xin-nong's Medical Record

Du, male, 15, first visit was on July 1, 1987

【Chief Complaint】
Enuresis for six years

【Present Medical History】
Six years ago the patient began to have enuresis. He would wet the bed less frequently in summer and more so during the winter. During the daytime, his urinary output was not large, it was white in colour, there was no low back pain. His appetite, sleep, memory, and bowel movement were normal.

【Examination】
Emaciation, sallow complexion, pale tongue with toothmarks and a thin yellow coating, thready weak pulse.

【Diagnosis】
Enuresis (due to spleen kidney yang deficiency)

【Treatment Principles】
Warm and reinforce spleen and kidney yang, strengthen qi to hold urine

【Treatment】

DU 20 (*bǎi huì*)	RN 6 (*qì hǎi*)	RN 4 (*guān yuán*)

ST 36 (*zú sān lǐ*)

SP 6 (*sān yīn jiāo*)	BL 23 (*shèn shù*)	BL 20 (*pí shù*)

Moxibustion was applied at RN 4 (*guān yuán*). BL 20 (*pí shù*) and BL 23 (*shèn shù*) were needled without retention of needles; all the other points were tonfied.

After four treatments, he would wake and get up to urinate. In order to consolidate the good result, acupuncture was continued for another 12 treatments and he was cured.

〖Note〗

Systematic Classic of Acupuncture - Moxibustion (Zhēn Jiǔ Jiǎ Yǐ Jīng, 针灸甲乙经) says: "Deficiency causes enuresis." The kidney dominates storage and controls qi activities; the urinary bladder is the organ to store and discharge urine; it depends on the warmth and nourishment of the kidney yang. If the kidney qi is deficient, the bladder will be deficient and cold and fail to control the water passages, thus enuresis occurs. In this boy's case the spleen is deficient, it fails to produce qi and blood, the muscles and skin lack nourishment, thus the emaciation and sallow complexion. Because the yang is deficient, there is a pale tongue with toothmarks, aversion to cold and a thready and weak pulse.

DU 20 (*bǎi huì*) is an intersecting point of the *du* vessel with all the yang channels, it rises the clear to bring up the sinking, and opens the orifices to benefit the brain. RN 4 (*guān yuán*) and RN 6 (*qì hǎi*) warm and tonify kidney yang which controls the qi transformation of the bladder. SP 6 (*sān yīn jiāo*) is an intersecting point of the three foot yin channels, regulates and tonifies the spleen and kidney. BL 23 (*shèn shù*) and BL 20 (*pí shù*) tonify spleen and kidney.

Yang Yong-xuan's Medical Record

Jin, male, 16

【Chief Complaint】

Enuresis since he was small.

【Present Medical History】

The patient would wet the bed two to three times each night

【Examination】

Moist tongue, slow but forceful pulse

【Diagnosis】

Enuresis (due to instability of the bladder qi)

【Treatment Principles】

Remove obstructions and tonify qi

【Treatment】

RN 4 (*guān yuán*)	SP 6 (*sān yīn jiāo*)

Rotating method. RN 4 (*guān yuán*) was tonified while SP 6 (*sān yīn jiāo*) drained. Treatment was given once every other day. After 10 treatments he would sometimes get up at night to urinate, but still occasionally had enuresis; as his lower *jiao* was deficient, he could not control his urine. The spleen and kidney were warmed and tonified, so now SP 6 (*sān yīn jiāo*) was also treated with a tonifying method. Four more treatments given once every other day basically cured him. The follow-up found no recurrence.

【Note】

Enuresis is intractable and difficult to treat and the causative factors are complex. Acupuncture is an effective treatment for it. In fact, all patients can be cured if they do not get overtired during the daytime and not drink too much water before going to bed in the evening, and are woken to pass water regularly at night.

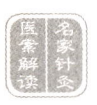

Summary

Enuresis refers to the urination at night without self-awareness. As written in the *Systematic Classic of Acupuncture - Moxibustion* "Deficiency causes enuresis". Enuresis is of qi deficiency. For treatment, the principle is to tonify and augment kidney qi to strengthen the qi transformation of the bladder.

Main points: RN 4 (*guān yuán*) and SP 6 (*sān yīn jiāo*).

Add HT 7 (*shén mén*) for those who are fuzzy headed before urinating. Needle DU 20 (*bǎi huì*) for those who have frequent urination. Add BL 23 (*shèn shù*) and BL 28 (*páng guāng shù*) for those who are weak in constitution due to prolonged disease.

Zhà Sāi (MUMPS)

Cheng Xin-nong's Medical Record

Shi, female, 46, first visit was on April 7, 1980

【Chief Complaint】

The left parotid region was painful and swollen for five days

【Present Medical History】

Five days ago, the patient had pain and swelling in the left mandible region, three days ago it spread to the whole mandible region. She had a slight fever, body temperature was 37.8℃(100℉). Now the left parotid region was swollen and painful, with paroxysmal pain on the left side. She had some vomiting from taking anti-inflammatory medication. She also had a slight cough, her appetite was almost normal.

【Examination】

Pale red tongue, white dry coating, thready rolling pulse

【Diagnosis】

Mumps (*Zhà Sāi*) (due to invasion of epidemic pathogen)

【Treatment Principles】

Regulate the *shaoyang* channel, transform the accumulation, stop pain

【Treatment】

DU 14 (*dà zhuī*)	SJ 5 (*wài guān*)	LI 4 (*hé gǔ*)
Left side:	SJ 17 (*yì fēng*)	ST 6 (*jiá chē*)
	SI 17 (*tiān róng*)	

Even method. After the first acupuncture treatment, her pain was relieved. With five treatments, her mumps were cured.

【Note】

The invasion of exogenous epidemic pathogenic heat blocks the *shaoyang* channel, obstructing the qi of this channel, thus the pain. The points are mainly selected from the local area and the affected *shaoyang* channel to regulate its qi circulation and remove obstruction to stop pain.

Summary

Mumps, also known as *Há Ma Wēn* (蛤蟆瘟), is an acute infectious disease caused by exogenous epidemic pathogenic heat, which manifests as fever, swelling and pain in the parotid region. It is mostly seen in children but sometimes also in adults. In modern medicine, it is called epidemic parotitis. In some children, it causes lower abdominal pain and testicle pain.

Main points: SJ 17 (*yì fēng*), ST 6 (*jiá chē*), LI 4 (*hé gǔ*).

Add LI 11 (*qū chí*) and SJ 5 (*wài guān*) for fever.

For severe swelling and pain, bleed LU 11 (*shào shāng*) and LI 1 (*shāng yáng*).

Add RN 3 (*zhōng jí*), SP 6 (*sān yīn jiāo*) and LV 3 (*tài chōng*) if there is accompanying testitis.

CHAPTER **3** **DISEASES OF EYES, EARS, NOSE AND THROAT**

Internal Diseases

Gynecological and
Pediatric Diseases

Diseases of Eyes,
Ears, Nose and
Throat

Skin Diseases,
External Diseases

Others

TINNITUS AND DEAFNESS

Cheng Xin-nong's Medical Record

Shi, male, 62, first visit was on February 25, 1982

【Chief Complaint】
Loss of hearing in the left ear for three months

【Present Medical History】
Three months ago, the patient had a common cold, which affected the hearing of his left ear and was accompanied by tinnitus. He went to the Beijing Tongren Hospital for an examination that found him to have a sunken tympanic membrane; he was diagnosed with sudden deafness of the left ear. He often had a dry mouth and dream-disturbed sleep.

【Examination】
BP 150/90 mm Hg. Pale flabby tongue with toothmarks, wiry and slippery pulse.

【Diagnosis】
Sudden deafness (due to phlegm fire disturbing upward)

【Treatment Principles】
Remove obstruction from the ear, clear fire, transform phlegm

【Treatment】

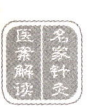

DU 20 (*bǎi huì*)	GB 20 (*fēng chí*)	SJ 5 (*wài guān*)
LI 4 (*hé gǔ*)	SJ 3 (*zhōng zhǔ*)	GB 34 (*yáng líng quán*)
SP 6 (*sān yīn jiāo*)	LV 3 (*tài chōng*)	
Left side:	SJ 17 (*yì fēng*)	SI 19 (*tīng gōng*)

Even method. On March 1, 1982 he came again. RN 12 (*zhōng wǎn*) and ST 36 (*zú sān lǐ*) were added to the treatment. The hearing of his left ear was greatly improved.

【Note】

The gallbladder channel runs up to the corner of the forehead and down to the back of the ear, where it enters into the brain. Phlegm and damp are brought upward by the liver and gall bladder fire and attack the ear, causing the sudden deafness.

DU 20 (*bǎi huì*) is selected to regulate yin and yang as well as qi and blood. GB 20 (*fēng chí*), SI 19 (*tīng gōng*) and SJ 17 (*yì fēng*) remove obstructions from the ear. SJ 5 (*wài guān*) and SJ 3 (*zhōng zhǔ*) circulate the qi of the *shaoyang* channel. LV 3 (*tài chōng*) and LI 4 (*hé gǔ*) move qi and invigorate the blood to remove obstructions. ST 36 (*zú sān lǐ*), SP 6 (*sān yīn jiāo*) and RN 12 (*zhōng wǎn*) strengthen the spleen and harmonize the stomach, transform phlegm and damp. GB 34 (*yáng líng quán*) relaxes the wood and strengthens the earth.

Xiao Shao-qing's Medical Record

Fan, male, 60, first visit was on October 25, 1994

【Chief Complaint】

Loss of hearing of the right ear for two years

【Present Medical History】

This patient's wife died after which he suffered from severe depression. He suddenly started to experience dizziness accompanied by tinnitus and a decline of hearing and then a loss of hearing. Gulou Hospital diagnosed him with sudden deafness. Medication was not helpful. At the time of his visit the hearing in his right ear was completely gone, and he felt an obstruction in the ear, especially on rainy days. This patient often experienced irritability. His sleep, appetite, urination and defecation were normal.

【Examination】

Pale red tongue with a white sticky coating, wiry and slippery pulse

【Diagnosis】

Deafness (due to liver qi bringing the phlegm upward to disturb the ear)

【Treatment Principles】

Calm the liver and regulate qi, strengthen the spleen and transform phlegm, remove obstructions from the ear, restore hearing

【Treatment】

LI 4 (*hé gŭ*)	ST 36 (*zú sān lǐ*)	SP 6 (*sān yīn jiāo*)
LV 3 (*tài chōng*)		
Right side:	GB 2 (*tīng huì*)	SJ 17 (*yì fēng*)
SJ 3 (*zhōng zhŭ*)		

Even method. Retaining the needles for 20 minutes and manipulating once every 10 minutes. After removing the needles, indirect moxibustion with ginger was applied at GB 2 (*tīng huì*), 5 cones were used till the skin became reddish. The patient was treated once a day.

After two treatments, he felt the tinnitus and obstruction was reduced. Professor Xiao thought this was a sign that the auditory nerve began to recover, so he changed the even method to a draining method to excite the auditory nerve and taught the patient to do Self-Blow of qi. After 11 treatments, the patient could distinguish the sound of music and speaking. One month's treatment helped him hear clearly.

【Note】

This patient was depressed and worried because of the death of his wife. Constraint from depression damages the liver and worry damages the spleen. There was liver qi stagnation and phlegm formed due to failure of the spleen in transportation and transformation. The liver qi brings the phlegm upward to disturb the ear, causing deafness. GB 2 (*tīng huì*) and SJ 17 (*yì fēng*) are local points for deafness. *Treatment of Diseases in Verse* says:

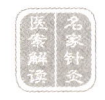

"For distention and obstruction in the ear GB 2 (*tīng huì*) and SJ 17 (*yì fēng*) are the points to treat." These two points regulate the qi of the *san jiao* and *shaoyang*. LI 4 (*hé gǔ*) and LV 3 (*tài chōng*) are the four gates, they strongly move qi and invigorate blood to calm the liver and relieve depression. ST 36 (*zú sān lǐ*) and SP 6 (*sān yīn jiāo*) strengthen spleen and stomach, transform phlegm and restore hearing. As for the techniques of needling, according to Professor Xiao, the local points should be needled deeply, otherwise the treatment is useless. So SJ 17 (*yì fēng*) and GB 2 (*tīng huì*) are inserted as deep as 1.5 inches. Indirect moxibustion with ginger at the local area can warm and remove obstruction from the channels, it is good for chronic cases and deficiency syndromes.

> **Self-Blow of** qi: *On getting up in the morning, after washing, the patient takes 10 or more deep breaths, then relaxes for 1~2 minutes, takes one deep inhalation, closes the mouth, pinches the nostrils closed, then blows the qi from eustachian tube into the ear till the tympanic membrane starts gurgling.*
>
> *It is used to balance the pressure inside and outside the ear to treat the sunken drum.*

Summary

Tinnitus and *deafness* are differentiated by excess and deficiency. The excess syndrome is caused by liver and gall bladder fire or phlegm fire rising upward to cause a disturbance, or by wind and heat invasion blocking the channel qi of the ears. The deficiency syndrome is caused by kidney qi deficiency, in this case either the essential qi is not ample enough to nourish the ear, or there is a sinking of qi in middle *jiao*, also causing a lack of nourishment. In the case of deafness due to injury from a trauma, the tongue coating and pulse can be normal, it is regarded as excess syndrome and treated accordingly.

Main points: SJ 17 (*yì fēng*), SJ 3 (*zhōng zhǔ*), SI 19 (*tīng gōng*) or SJ 21 (*ěr mén*) or GB 2 (*tīng huì*).

Add GB 20 (*fēng chí*) and LV 2 (*xíng jiān*) for liver and gall bladder fire. For phlegm fire upward disturbing add ST 40 (*fēng lóng*). BL 23 (*shèn shù*), KI 3 (*tài xī*) and RN 6 (*qì hǎi*) are used for kidney yin deficiency. Needle DU 20 (*bǎi huì*) to treat sinking of qi in the middle *jiao*. DU 14 (*dà zhuī*) and LI 4 (*hé gǔ*) are used for invasion of exogenous pathogenic factors.

CONGESTION, SWELLING AND PAIN OF THE EYE

Shao Jing-ming's Medical Record

Wang, female, 40, first visit was on May 20, 1992

【Chief Complaint】

Congestion, swelling and pain of the eyes for four days

【Present Medical History】

This patient's eyes were congested, swollen and painful; due to photophobia and lacrimation it was difficult for her to open them. She had blurred vision for four days already. Gentamycin intramuscular injection and chloromycetin eye drops did not help.

【Examination】

Swelling of the eyelids, seriously congested palpebral conjunctiva, big patches of bleeding at the bulbar conjunctiva on the temporal side of the eyeballs, and a large amount of sticky discharge. Red tongue, wiry rapid pulse.

【Diagnosis】

Congestion, swelling and pain of the eyes (due to hyperactivity of pathogenic heat)

【Treatment Principles】

Clear heat, remove toxins, relieve swelling, stop pain

【Treatment】

tài yáng (EX-HN5)	BL 2 (*cuán zhú*)	*ěr jiān* (EX-HN6)
Ear points:	Eye	liver

Tài yáng (EX-HN5) was bled (in case the bleeding is not enough, cupping with a small cup can be used to draw out more blood.) BL 2 (*cuán zhú*) and *ěr jiān* (EX-HN6) also were bled, as well as the ear points for the eye and liver.

After one bleeding treatment, the patient had a reduction in pain. On the following day the swelling and pain disappeared and congestion subsided. Two more bleeding treatments at *tài yáng* (EX-HN5), BL 2 (*cuán zhú*) and *ěr jiān* (EX-HN6) were done and she was cured.

【Note】

Bleeding is very effective in the treatment of eye diseases, such as acute conjunctivitis, keratitis, sties, corneal opacity, trachomas, and electric ophthalmia. Using a three-edged needle to bleed *tài yáng* (EX-HN5) can improve the blood circulation of eye tissues to dispel wind, invigorate blood, clear heat and promote vision. As written in the *Jade Dragon Verse*: "For the congestion, swelling and pain of the eyes with aversion to light, puncture BL 1 (*jīng míng*) and bleed *tài yáng* (EX-HN5) for a cure."

BL 2 (*cuán zhú*) functions to smooth the channel qi and dispel wind, clear heat, remove obstructions from the channels, and stop pain. *Ěr jiān* (EX-HN6) functions to reduce fever, treat inflammation, calm the mind and stop pain. The ear points: eye and liver have the functions to clear liver fire, cool blood and promote vision. This group of points is effective in clearing heat, removing toxins, relieving swelling, and stopping pain, they give good therapeutic results.

Summary

Congestion, swelling and pain of the eyes is involved in acute conjunctivitis, mostly seen in the spring and autumn, and accompanied by photophobia, lacrimation and sticky discharge. In those cases caused by invasion of wind heat, the accompanying symptoms will be headache, fever, and superficial rapid pulse; in the cases caused by liver and gall bladder fire, the accompanying symptoms will be a bitter taste in the mouth, irritability, and wiry pulse.

Main points: BL 1 (*jīng míng*), GB 20 (*fēng chí*), LI 4 (*hé gǔ*), and *tài yáng* (EX-HN5).

Bleed *tài yáng* (EX-HN5). Add LU 11 (*shào shāng*), LI 2 (*èr jiān*) and BL 2 (*cuán zhú*) for the wind heat syndrome. For liver and gall bladder fire use LV 3 (*tài chōng*) and needle *tài yáng* (EX-HN5) through to GB 8 (*shuài gǔ*).

BLURRED VISION

Cheng Xin-nong's Medical Record

Xu, male, 73, first visit was on May 16, 1992

【Chief Complaint】
Decline of vision in both eyes for four years

【Present Medical History】
In 1988, he was diagnosed with optic atrophy, he had blurred vision with a corrected vision 0.2. When he was tired, his blood pressure would be higher.

【Examination】
Greasy yellow coating, the left pulse was thready and wiry, the proximal pulse of both sides was weak

【Diagnosis】
Blurred vision (due to liver and kidney deficiency)

【Treatment Principles】
Reinforce the liver and kidney, replenish blood, promote vision

【Treatment】

DU 20 (*bǎi huì*)	ST 2 (*sì bái*)	GB 1 (*tóng zǐ liáo*)	SI 6 (*yǎng lǎo*)
PC 6 (*nèi guān*)	LI 4 (*hé gǔ*)	GB 37 (*guāng míng*)	SP 6 (*sān yīn jiāo*)

| KI 3 (*tài xī*) | LV 3 (*tài chōng*) | BL 17 (*gé shù*) | BL 18 (*gān shù*) |

BL 23 (*shèn shù*)

SP 6 (*sān yīn jiāo*), KI 3 (*tài xī*), BL 17 (*gé shù*), BL 18 (*gān shù*) and BL 23 (*shèn shù*) were tonified, other points were treated with an even method.

After four courses of treatment, the patient reported the eyes did not get tired so easily, and the blurred vision improved. After two more courses for consolidation, he could see clearly and he stopped treatment.

【Note】

The liver opens into the eyes, the kidney stores essence and dominates the pupils. This patient is elderly, his liver blood and kidney yin are deficient, thus unable to nourish the eyes, so he has blurred vision.

Summary

Blurred vision, a common disease in the elderly, is the result of yin and blood deficiency and weakness of the liver and kidney. The essential substances of the five *zang* and six *fu* organs pour up to nourish the eyes. With enough nourishment of blood, the eyes can see clearly, without enough blood for nourishment, there will be blurred vision. Therefore, tonifying the liver and kidney and replenishing blood to promote vision are the basic principles for treatment.

Commonly used points: BL 1 (*jīng míng*), ST 2 (*sì bái*), SI 6 (*yǎng lǎo*), GB 37 (*guāng míng*), LV 3 (*tài chōng*), BL 17 (*gé shù*), BL 18 (*gān shù*), and BL 23 (*shèn shù*). Use a tonifying method.

MYOPIA

Cheng Xin-nong's Medical Record

Ge, female, 31, first visit was on August 17, 1984

【Chief Complaint】

Decline of vision for 22 years, worse in the past four years

【Present Medical History】

Twenty-two years ago, this patient suffered from acute hepatitis. After it was cured, she noticed that her vision began to decline and gradually became worse. Tongren Hospital diagnosed her myopia. Four years ago after giving birth, her vision in both eyes was 0.1 and there were excess secretions. Appetite and sleep were normal.

【Examination】

Pale dark tongue with a thin white coating, thready pulse

【Diagnosis】

Myopia (due to liver blood deficiency)

【Treatment Principles】

Strengthen the spleen and tonify the liver, tonify deficiency and promote vision

【Treatment】

DU 20 (bǎi huì)	GB 20 (fēng chí)	BL 1 (jīng míng)	BL 2 (cuán zhú)	ST 2 (sì bái)
ST 36 (zú sān lǐ)	GB 37 (guāng míng)	SP 6 (sān yīn jiāo)	LV 3 (tài chōng)	

Tonifying method. After 70 treatments, her vision was greatly improved.

【Note】

The eyes are the organs of vision. Only with the nourishment of essential qi of the five *zang* and six *fu* organs can the vision be sharp. The liver opens into the eye, if the liver blood is deficient, the vision will decline.

Zhong Mei-quan's Medical Record

Xiao, male, 9

【Chief Complaint】

Poor distance vision for four years

【Present Medical History】

He could not see distant objects clearly, sometimes he had double vision and the eyes were easily fatigued. He had worn glasses for one year. In the past, he had a bad habit of reading at a very short distance. His appetite was good; urination and defecation were normal.

【Examination】

Examination showed the myopia of the right eye −1.50 and astigmatism +1.50; the myopia of the left eye −1.00 and astigmatism +0.75, and the corrected vision of both eyes 1.2. At both sides of the first cervical vertebra, there were nodules and rope-like objects felt along with tenderness. The tip of the tongue was red, coating thin, and pulse thready and wiry.

【Diagnosis】

Myopia (due to liver and kidney deficiency, heart blood deficiency)

【Treatment Principles】

Replenish heart blood, tonify liver and kidney

【Treatment】

zhèng guāng (Empirical point)	GB 20 (*fēng chí*)

After one course of treatment the sight in his right eye improved from 0.6 to 1.2 and left eye from 0.6 to 1.5.

In the second course, PC 6 (*nèi guān*) was added in treatment. The sight in both eyes improved to 1.5. The symptoms disappeared, he could see clearly with no need to use glasses. The treatment was stopped and he was asked to pay attention to protecting vision and to do self-massage at *zhèng guāng* point. A follow-up after seven years found that the vision of both eyes remained at 1.5.

【Note】

Myopia is common in teenagers. For treatment, in addition to filiform needle acupuncture, tapping with the plum-blossom needle is also applied. From observation of myopia cases those under the age of 20 with mild cases of myopia often had their vision restored to normal, while more than 50% of those with more serious cases had remarkable improvement in their vision.

Main points:	zhèng guāng	zhèng guāng₂	
Accompanying points:	GB 20 (fēng chí)	PC 6 (nèi guān)	DU 14 (dà zhuī)
	BL 15 (xīn shù)	BL 18 (gān shù)	BL 19 (dǎn shù)
	BL 23 (shèn shù)		

Tapping: Tap with the plum-blossom hammer 20~50 times within 0.5~1.2 cm of the point you wish to treat. Once every other day, 15 treatments is one course, half a month for rest, and continue the treatment if necessary. Within half a year to one year, the patient should be re-examined and treated once every half a month to one month to consolidate the therapeutic effect.

Zhèng guāng (Empirical point) is located at the junction of the lateral 3/4 and medial 1/4 of the supraorbital margin, namely between BL 2 (*cuán zhú*) and *yú yāo* (EX-HN4), inferior to the supraorbital margin.

Zhèng guāng₂ (Empirical point) is located at the junction of the lateral 1/4 and medial 3/4 of the supraorbital margin, namely between SJ 23 (*sī zhú kōng*) and *yú yāo* (EX-HN4), inferior to the supraorbital margin.

The selection of above-mentioned points was based on the theory that the liver opens into the eye. *Zhèng guāng* and *zhèng guāng₂* (Empirical points) function to replenish blood, tonify the liver, and promote vision. GB 20 (*fēng chí*), due to its external/internal relationship with the liver is effective in calming the liver, clearing the mind and promoting vision. PC 6 (*nèi guān*), the *luò*-connecting point of the pericardium channel of hand *juéyīn*, activates heart yang and replenishes heart blood. DU 14 (*dà zhuī*) regulates qi and blood, strengthens the body and tonifies yang. BL 15 (*xīn shù*), BL 18 (*gān shù*), BL 19 (*dǎn shù*), and BL 23 (*shèn shù*) remove the obstructions from the channel. BL 15 (*xīn shù*) unobstructs heart qi and replenishes heart blood; BL 18 (*gān shù*) and BL 19 (*dǎn shù*) calm the liver and gall bladder, replenish blood and tonify the liver; BL 23 (*shèn shù*)

tonifies the kidney and promotes kidney yang.

Summary

Myopia is an eye disease of ametropia, caused by improper usage of eyes in reading in a dim light or due to heredity factors.

Main points: ST 1 (*chéng qì*), BL 1 (*jīng míng*), GB 20 (*fēng chí*), *yì míng* (EX-HN14), and GB 37 (*guāng míng*).

BL 23 (*shèn shù*) and ST 36 (*zú sān lǐ*) are added for those who have chronic illness or a weak constitution.

Yì míng (EX-HN14) is located one inch posterior to SJ 17 (*yì fēng*), it is indicated for eye diseases, such as myopia, hyperopia, early stage cataracts, headache, dizziness, and tinnitus.

VISUAL FATIGUE

Record in *Acupuncture - Moxibustion for Difficult Diseases* (*Qí Nán Zá Bìng Zhēn Jiǔ Zhì Liáo*)

Fan, female, 28, first visit was on November 13, 1999

[Chief Complaint]

Mild blurred vision for four months

[Present Medical History]

This patient was engaged in mental work for a long time and very often worked overtime. Due to eyestrain she had blurred vision and visual fatigue. She was listless with poor appetite and slept poorly.

[Examination]

Pale tongue, white coating, thready weak pulse

[Diagnosis]

Visual fatigue (due to liver blood deficiency)

【Treatment Principles】

Regulate qi and blood, calm the mind, promote vision

【Treatment】

BL 1 (*jīng míng*)	ST 1 (*chéng qì*)	LV 3 (*tài chōng*)
ST 36 (*zú sān lǐ*)	SP 6 (*sān yīn jiāo*)	PC 6 (*nèi guān*)

Treatment was given once a day. After five treatments her condition improved. Another five treatments cured her.

【Note】

This patient's visual fatigue resulted from long term eyestrain and blood deficiency. TCM holds that eyes can see clearly only with enough blood nourishment. ST 36 (*zú sān lǐ*), SP 6 (*sān yīn jiāo*) and LV 3 (*tài chōng*) tonify the liver, spleen and kidney and regulate qi and blood. BL 1 (*jīng míng*) and ST 1 (*chéng qì*) regulate qi of the channels in the local region. PC 6 (*nèi guān*) relaxes the chest to regulate qi, settles the heart and calms the mind.

Bí Yuān (RHINORRHEA)

Cheng Xin-nong's Medical Records

Wu, male, 25, first visit was on January 19, 1982

【Chief Complaint】

Yellow nasal discharge for more than 10 years

【Present Medical History】

This patient was diagnosed with nasosinusitis, previous treatment was not satisfactory.

【Examination】

Thin tongue coating, slightly slow pulse

【Diagnosis】

Rhinorrhea (*Bí Yuān*) (due to stagnant heat in lung channel)

【Treatment Principles】

Dispel wind, clear heat, promote diffusion of the lung, remove obstruction of the nose

【Treatment】

BL 7 (*tōng tiān*)	DU 23 (*shàng xīng*)	*shàng yíng xiāng* (EX-HN8)
LI 20 (*yíng xiāng*)	LI 4 (*hé gǔ*)	LU 7 (*liè quē*)

Draining method. Twenty treatments greatly relieved his symptoms.

【Note】

The lung dominates qi and respiration, upward it connects with the trachea and the throat and opens into the nose; outward it correspond to the skin and skin hair. The appearance of *Bí Yuān* is closely related to the invasion of the lung channel by pathogenic factors. Wind cold attacks the lung and later transforms into fire, the lung loses its function in dispersing, thus causing obstruction of nose. Although wind cold is driven off, the heat is not cleared out, thus drying the fluid into a turbid mess and blocking the nose.

BL 7 (*tōng tiān*) acts to dispel wind, clear heat and open the nose. DU 23 (*shàng xīng*) and LI 20 (*yíng xiāng*) are the local points to unobstruct the nose. *Shàng yíng xiāng* (EX-HN8) is an important point for nose diseases, having an immediate effect on sneezing as it opens the nose. LI 4 (*hé gǔ*) and LU 7 (*liè quē*), a powerful combination of *yuán* - source and *luò* - connecting points, promote diffusion of the lung to open the nose.

> *Shàng yíng xiāng* (EX-HN8) is located on the face, at the junction of the nasal alar cartilage and nasal conchae, close to the upper portion of the nasolabial groove. It clears heat, unobstructs the nose, and is indicated for headache, nasal obstruction and lacrimation.

Li, female, 55, first visit was on November 16, 1991

【Chief Complaint】

Nasal obstruction with thick and sticky discharge for seven years

【Present Medical History】

This patient had nasal obstruction with thick and sticky discharge for seven years; treatment by Chinese and western medicine was not very effective. She had a dark complexion, her nose was obstructed with thick and sticky discharge that was made worse with repeated exposure to cold or without obvious reasons. She had coughing with an aversion to cold, lacrimation, and wheezing when the attack was serious.

【Examination】

Tongue tip was red, coating thick sticky and yellow in the middle, pulse wiry, proximal position weak.

【Diagnosis】

Rhinorrhea (*Bí Yuān*) (due to stagnated heat in lung and gall bladder)

【Treatment Principles】

Clear heat, transform phlegm, unobstruct the nose

【Treatment】

DU 14 (*dà zhuī*)	GB 20 (*fēng chí*)	LI 20 (*yíng xiāng*)	BL 7 (*tōng tiān*)	
DU 23 (*shàng xīng*)	LI 4 (*hé gǔ*)	LU 7 (*liè quē*)	KI 3 (*tài xī*)	LV 3 (*tài chōng*)

Draining method. After six treatments the aversion to cold, lacrimation, nasal obstruction with thick and sticky discharge were better. After 12 treatments all the symptoms were much improved, so she stopped coming.

【Note】

Simple Questions - On the Diseases due to Intertransference of Cold and Heat Evils Between Various Organs (*Sù Wèn: Qì Jué Lùn*, 素问 • 气厥论) says: "Heat from the gall bladder moving to the brain, there will be tingling in the nose with thick and sticky discharge." Thus stagnated heat in the gall bladder channel is one of the causative factors of *Bí Yuān*.

Record in *Acupuncture - Moxibustion for Difficult Diseases* (*Qí Nán Zá Bìng Zhēn Jiŭ Zhì Liáo*)

Xia, male, 28, first visit was on November 8, 1999

【Chief Complaint】

Runny nose in the morning and evening for one year

【Present Medical History】

This patient had a runny and itchy nose in the morning and evening, aversion to cold, and easily came down with the common cold. He was diagnosed with allergic rhinitis and was treated in the ENT department with anti-allergic drugs, but it was not effective.

【Examination】

Pale tongue, white coating, thready pulse

【Diagnosis】

Rhinorrhea (*Bí Yuān*) (due to wind cold attacking the lung)

【Treatment Principles】

Promote diffusion of the lung, remove obstructions from the nose

【Treatment】

LI 4 (*hé gŭ*)	LI 20 (*yíng xiāng*)	DU 24 (*shén tíng*)
BL 13 (*fèi shù*)	BL 20 (*pí shù*)	DU 25 (*sù liáo*)

Moxibustion was applied to BL 13 (*fèi shù*) and BL 20 (*pí shù*). DU 25 (*sù liáo*) was needled through to *yìn táng* (EX-HN3).

After five treatments, the symptoms were reduced, another five treatments and all the symptoms disappeared. His colds were also reduced in frequency. A four month follow up failed to find any reoccurrence.

【Note】

LI 4 (*hé gǔ*), LI 20 (*yíng xiāng*), DU 25 (*sù liáo*) and DU 24 (*shén tíng*) are the first choice points for nose diseases. BL 13 (*fèi shù*) and BL 20 (*pí shù*) are the back-shu points from where the qi of the lung and spleen are infused. Moxibustion can clear heat from the lung and transform phlegm, as well as strengthen the spleen to transform damp.

Summary

Rhinorrhea (*Bí Yuān*, thick and sticky nasal discharge) is caused by wind cold invading the lung, transforming into heat and obstructing the nose; or the damp heat of the gall bladder channel rises upward and blocks the nose. For treatment, points are mainly selected from the hand *taiyin* lung channel and the hand *yangming* large intestine channel to promote the lung in dispersing and clearing heat. Acupuncture is applied with a draining method.

Main points: DU 23 (*shàng xīng*), LI 20 (*yíng xiāng*), LI 4 (*hé gǔ*), and LU 7 (*liè quē*).

GB 20 (*fēng chí*) and BL 11 (*dà zhù*) are used for nasal obstruction. BL 13 (*fèi shù*) and LU 9 (*tài yuān*) used to treat thin, white nasal discharge. DU 14 (*dà zhuī*), LU 5 (*chǐ zé*) and LU 11 (*shào shāng*) are effective for yellow bloody discharge and fever. *Tài yáng* (EX-HN5) and *yìn táng* (EX-HN3) are added for headache.

SORE THROAT

Yang Yong-xuan's Medical Record

Chen, female, 21

【Chief Complaint】

Sore throat for three days

【Present Medical History】

This patient had acute pharyngolaryngitis for three days; was treated with western drugs and felt a little better. Since yesterday she had a hoarse voice, seriously sore throat with yellow thick phlegm and difficulty breathing.

【Examination】

The tongue coating was thin and dry, pulse thready and rapid

【Diagnosis】

Acute pharyngolaryngitis (due to invasion of wind heat)

【Treatment Principles】

Clear heat, transform phlegm, promote the lung in dispersing

【Treatment】

RN 22 (*tiān tū*)	PC 6 (*nèi guān*)	LI 4 (*hé gǔ*)	KI 3 (*tài xī*)

The rotating method for tonifying and draining was adopted. RN 22 (*tiān tū*) was treated without retention of the needle. Other points were treated with the needles being retained for 10 minutes.

On the 5th treatment, she already had much of the pain reduced and could speak with a clear voice, but still had an itchy throat. Since the phlegm was not yet transformed, RN 23 (*lián quán*) was added to regulate qi and remove obstruction of the nose. RN 23 (*lián quán*) was drained without retaining the needle. All the symptoms disappeared and she was cured.

【Note】

The acute pharyngolaryngitis, known as sore throat, is mostly caused by an invasion of wind heat burning the throat, or overwork with deficiency fire flaring up to the throat. In a mild case, the patient feels dryness and pain in the throat; in serious cases there will be a difficulty in swallowing, and chills and fever. This patient has a mild case, her sore throat is due to exogenous pathogenic heat flaring upward and exhaustion of the body fluids of the lung transforming into phlegm heat.

RN 22 (*tiān tū*) is selected to promote the lung in dispersing and transforming phlegm. PC 6 (*nèi guān*) circulates qi in the chest. LI 4 (*hé gǔ*) clears heat from the lung. KI 3 (*tài xī*) is tonified to clear the voice and relieve the sore throat. In addition, an empirical point, *lì yān* (EX-HN21), is treated with an even method for a sore throat. Most of the patients will have their pain relieved within one hour after needling and be well on their way to recovery within five to six hours.

> *Lì yān (EX-HN21), located 0.8 inch lateral to LI 17 (tiān dǐng), it is needled to a depth of 0.5~1.0 inch. It is indicated for acute pharyngolaryngitis, acute tonsillitis, and hoarse voice.*

Cheng Xin-nong's Medical Records

Zhang, female, 21, first visit was on September 27, 1984

【Chief Complaint】
Dry throat for five years

【Present Medical History】
Five years ago, this patient began to have dry throat for no obvious reason. Diagnosed pharyngitis in Youdian Hospital, she was administered western drugs, but it was not effective. Now she has a dry, sore throat and hoarse voice; it is made worse by intake of spicy food.

【Examination】
Pale dark tongue with cracks, thready pulse

【Diagnosis】
Dry throat (due to yin deficiency of lung and kidney)

【Treatment Principles】
Replenish yin, moisten throat

【Treatment】

LU 7 (*liè quē*)	KI 3 (*tài xī*)	KI 6 (*zhào hǎi*)
LI 4 (*hé gǔ*)	SP 6 (*sān yīn jiāo*)	LI 17 (*tiān dǐng*)

[Note]

Yān (pharynx) connects with the esophagus, leading to the stomach, while *Hóu* (larynx) connects with the trachea, leading to the lung. The exhaustion of essential qi of the lung and kidney causes deficiency fire that flaring upward gives rise to throat dryness. KI 3 (*tài xī*) is the *yuán*-source point of the foot *shaoyin* kidney channel, KI 6 (*zhào hǎi*) opens the *yinqiao mai*, together they replenish yin to subdue the fire; bringing down the deficiency fire being the important principle for treating dry throat. SP 6 (*sān yīn jiāo*) strengthens, while KI 3 (*tài xī*) and KI 6 (*zhào hǎi*) replenish yin to subdue the fire. LU 7 (*liè quē*), the *luò*-connecting point of the hand *taiyin*, LI 4 (*hé gǔ*), the *yuán*-source of the hand *yangming*, and LI 17 (*tiān dǐng*), a point of the hand *yangming*, used together clear the stagnated heat of the *taiyin* and *yangming* channels.

Yao, male, 29, first visit was on May 19, 1992

[Chief Complaint]

Sore throat for half a year

[Present Medical History]

The patient was diagnosed with chronic pharyngitis. Treatment with Chinese and western medicine did not relieve his symptoms. He had a dry and sore throat, numbness of the tongue, dry lips, ulcers in the mouth, insomnia, listlessness, fatigue, and low back pain.

[Examination]

Swollen tonsils, red tongue with cracks, toothmarks on borders, sparse coating, wiry pulse, proximal position weak

[Diagnosis]

Sore throat (yin deficiency of lung and kidney)

[Treatment Principles]

Reinforce lung and kidney, replenish yin, subdue fire

【Treatment】

LI 17 (tiān dǐng)	LI 11 (qū chí)	LU 7 (liè quē)	LU 10 (yú jì)	LI 4 (hé gǔ)
HT 7 (shén mén)	SP 6 (sān yīn jiāo)	KI 3 (tài xī)	KI 6 (zhào hǎi)	

SP 6 (sān yīn jiāo), KI 3 (tài xī) and KI 6 (zhào hǎi) were tonified, LI 11 (qū chí) was drained, other points were treated with an even method.

After eight treatments the sore throat was relieved and he could sleep. Two courses of treatment pretty much cleared up his problem.

【Note】

Yin deficiency of lung and kidney leads to deficiency fire flaring up, causing dry, sore throat and insomnia. The low back pain, fatigue and constipation are due to deficiency of kidney water.

Summary

Sore throat, known as *Hóu Bì* (喉痹) in TCM, is divided into deficiency and excess syndromes. The excess case is from the invasion of exogenous pathogenic wind heat burning the lung, or stagnated heat of the lung and stomach channels harassing upward; the deficiency case is from yin deficiency of the kidney causing the deficiency fire flaring up.

For excess syndrome, the points are mainly selected from the hand and foot *yangming* channels to dispel wind heat, they are needled with a draining method.

Main points: LU 11 (*shào shāng*), LI 4 (*hé gǔ*), ST 44 (*nèi tíng*), and SI 17 (*tiān róng*).

For deficiency syndrome, the points are mainly selected from the foot *shaoyin* kidney channel to replenish yin and subdue fire, they are needled with a tonifying method.

Main points: KI 3 (*tài xī*), LU 10 (*yú jì*), SP 6 (*sān yīn jiāo*), KI 6 (*zhào hǎi*), and LU 7 (*liè quē*).

TOOTHACHE

Yang Jie-bin's Medical Record

Duo, male, 23, first visit was on December 28, 1996

【Chief Complaint】
Toothache for seven days

【Present Medical History】
Seven days before his visit the patient began to have a toothache, which recently became worse. Now his on-again off-again tooth pain caused him to be unable to eat or sleep; he also had dizziness, chills and fever. Taking over the counter pain medication was of no use. His urine was yellow and stools dry.

【Examination】
Swollen gums and cheeks, bad breath, dental caries in the lower right pre-molar. Dry red tongue, thin yellow coating, superficial rapid pulse.

【Diagnosis】
Wind fire toothache (due to tooth decay)

【Treatment Principles】
Clear heat, reduce fire, dispel wind, stop pain

【Treatment】

ST 6 (*jiá chē*)	ST 5 (*dà yíng*)	LI 4 (*hé gǔ*)
ST 44 (*nèi tíng*)	*ā shì* (local points)	

The three-edged needle was used to bleed the *ā shì* (local points). Other points were treated with a strongly draining method. The heavy, distended sore needling sensation was a must! The needles were removed after the pain stopped. The needles were strongly stimulated once very three minutes during the time they were retained.

Ten minutes after insertion, the pain was relieved and after 30 minutes the pain stopped. On the following day the toothache returned and was treated as before twice more, after which the gum's swelling and pain disappeared.

【Note】

Hand and foot *yangming* channels distribute to the teeth. ST 6 (*jiá chē*) and ST 5 (*dà yíng*) are the local points used to remove obstructions from the channels and collaterals. LI 4 (*hé gǔ*) is a distal point that dispels wind to stop pain. ST 44 (*nèi tíng*) is a *Ying* - spring point to send the qi of the *fu* organs downward; it clears the stomach heat.

Sheng Xie-sun and Ling Xu-zhi's Medical Record

Jiang, male, 31, first visit was on June 20, 1960

【Chief Complaint】

Swelling and painful gums for five days

【Present Medical History】

After overindulging in spicy food five days ago, this patient's decayed teeth began to act up with cutting pain and gum swelling. The over the counter pain-killers were useless, filling the tooth was only effective for a little while. He was also constipated.

【Examination】

Tongue coating was yellow sticky and thick, proximal pulse surging.

【Diagnosis】

Toothache (stomach fire toothache)

【Treatment Principle】

Clear stomach heat to stop pain

【Treatment】

Left side:	LI 2 (èr jiān)	Right side:	ST 5 (dà yíng)

Draining method. Retaining needles for 20 minutes relieved the pain.

Sharp pain again returned in the afternoon, so he returned for treatment. LI 4 (hé gǔ) and ST 6 (jiá chē) were treated with a draining method, but the pain could not be controlled.

On the following day, LI 4 (hé gǔ), LI 6 (piān lì), ST 40 (fēng lóng) and ST 45 (lì duì) (left) were treated with a draining method; the needles were retained for 40 minutes and manipulated once every five minutes. This stopped the pain. The same treatment was given twice over the next two days, his tongue coating changed to normal and the pain was cured.

【Note】

In the first and second treatments the two groups of empirical points, LI 2 (èr jiān) and ST 5 (dà yíng) along with LI 4 (hé gǔ) and ST 6 (jiá chē) were used, but were not effective. In the third treatment, LI 4 (hé gǔ), LI 6 (piān lì), ST 40 (fēng lóng) and ST 45 (lì duì) were effectively used to relieve pain. This is because for excess heat syndromes due to yangming stomach fire flaming up, the principle "for the channel qi excess, reduce the collateral fullness" should be followed, therefore LI 6 (piān lì) and ST 40 (fēng lóng), the luò-connecting points of the hand and foot yangming were used to dredge the obstructed channels to subdue the stomach fire. This is also a proven experience of what is said in Lyrics of Standard Profoundities (Biāo Yōu Fù, 标幽赋): "Reduce the collateral with distal points, puncture the foot for diseases of the head."

Chen Zuo-lin's Medical Record

Huang, female, 68, first visit was on October 26, 1987

【Chief Complaint】

Gum pain for half a month

【Present Medical History】

This patient had gum pain that was worse in the afternoon and when she was tired.

【Examination】

No decayed teeth, no redness and swelling of gums, red tongue tip, without coating, thready rapid pulse.

【Diagnosis】

Toothache (due to yin deficiency, fire flaring up)

【Treatment Principles】

Nourish yin, tonify kidney, subdue fire, stop pain

【Treatment】

KI 3 (*tài xī*)

Three acupuncture treatments stopped the pain.

【Note】

Her pain is due to yin deficiency with deficient fire flaring up, so it was worse in the afternoon and when tired. KI 3 (*tài xī*) was selected to nourish yin and tonify the kidney to stop the fire from flaring up, thus the pain was stopped.

Summary

Toothache is a common disease that can be due to excess or deficiency fire. The excess toothache is caused by stomach heat and invasion of wind heat; it is called wind fire toothache. The deficiency toothache is the result of kidney yin-deficiency with deficient fire flaring up.

Main points: LI 4 (*hé gǔ*), ST 6 (*jiá chē*), and ST 7 (*xià guān*).

GB 20 (*fēng chí*) and ST 44 (*nèi tíng*) are added for wind fire syndrome; KI 3 (*tài xī*) is added for deficiency fire.

CHAPTER **4** **SKIN DISEASES, EXTERNAL DISEASES**

Internal Diseases

Gynecological and Pediatric Diseases

Diseases of Eyes, Ears, Nose and Throat

Skin Diseases, External Diseases

Others

ERYSIPELAS

Lu Shou-yan's Medical Record

Xu, female, 45, first visit was on July 1948

【Chief Complaint】

Redness, swelling and pain of the right leg and foot for three days

【Present Medical History】

Her right leg and foot was red and swollen with a hot sensation and severe pain.

【Examination】

The tongue coating was normal, the pulse soft and rapid

【Diagnosis】

Flowing fire (*Liú Huǒ*) (due to accumulated heat transformed into fire)

【Treatment Principles】

Clear heat, remove toxins

【Treatment】

BL 40 (*wěi zhōng*)	GB 34 (*yáng líng quán*)	BL 57 (*chéng shān*)
ST 36 (*zú sān lǐ*)	ST 40 (*fēng lóng*)	

Lifting-thrusting draining method was applied. BL 40 (*wěi zhōng*) was bled. The pain was relieved after the first treatment. Seven treatments cured her.

【Note】

Erysipelas is caused by an accumulation of heat that transforms into fire that then flows into the leg. This kind of swelling and pain, which is due to an obstruction of the channels, should be treated by removing toxic heat from the affected area; treat by using distal points of the affected channels. Bleeding BL 40 (*wěi zhōng*) removes toxic heat from the blood of the lower extremities.

Summary

Erysipelas is due to wind with accumulated damp heat infecting first the blood and then the skin and muscles. When on the leg, it is called flowing fire (*Liú Huǒ*流火) or Fire sores (*Huǒ Dān*火丹); when appearing on the face, it is called *Bào Tóu Huǒ Dān* (抱头火丹); when it involves the hypochondriac, lumbar and hip regions, it is called *Chì Yóu Dān* (赤游丹). This is an acute contagious infectious skin disease characterized by sudden onset of chills, fever, local redness and swelling which may affect any part of the body and rapidly expand to other areas. In chronic cases involving the legs that become thick and swollen, it is called *Dà Jiǎo Fēng* (大脚风).

Treat locally by surrounding the affected area with several shallowly inserted needles; blood-letting and cupping are used for removing the toxic heat.

Add DU 14 (*dà zhuī*), LI 11 (*qū chí*) and LI 4 (*hé gǔ*) for chills and fever. For high fever and thirst, bleed BL 40 (*wěi zhōng*) and *shí xuān* (EX-UE11). For headache needle *tài yáng* (EX-HN5) and GB 20 (*fēng chí*).

NAIL-LIKE BOIL

Peng Jing-shan's Medical Records

Tian, female, 22, first visit was on January 20, 1961.

【Chief Complaint】
Swelling and redness at the tip of the right middle finger

【Present Medical History】
Yesterday in the evening the patient noticed that there was swelling and

redness near the nail. The following morning it was worse as the colour changed from fresh red to blue purple and had a white pus filled top. Pain radiated down the medial side of forearm to the elbow; the pain was unendurable. She had chills and nausea.

【Examination】

Clear consciousness, sallow complexion, normal voice and respiration, thin white tongue coating, thready rapid pulse.

【Diagnosis】

Nail-like boil (*Dīng Dú*)

【Treatment】

Right side:	PC 1 (*tiān chí*)

The tonifying method using the rotating method caused the pain to stop immediately. A sharp round needle (Yuán Lì Zhēn 圆利针) was used to prick along the red line of inflammation up to the boil, the pain was relieved. The nausea and chills stopped as well.

On January 26, she came again and was cured.

【Note】

The boil at the tip of middle finger involved the pericardium channel. PC 1 (*tiān chí*) of the affected side was selected based on the head-tail treatment principle. Her pulse was thready rapid due to deficient heat, so a tonifying needling method was used.

Li, female, 40, first visit was on October 9, 1972

【Chief Complaint】

Numbness of the left palm for half a day

【Present Medical History】

This morning the patient felt numbness and pain of her left hand, chills, irritability and nausea.

【Examination】

Pale complexion, emaciation, and swelling of the left hand around HT 8 (*shào fǔ*) with a dull sensation, no change in skin colour. Red tongue, yellow coating, thready rapid pulse.

【Diagnosis】

Nail-like boil (*Dīng Dú*)

【Treatment】

HT 1 (*jí quán*)

Reinforcing method. The needle was retained for two minutes.

Her pain, cold feeling in the body and nausea disappeared. She said she felt very comfortable after needling.

【Note】

The boil in the region of HT 8 (*shào fǔ*), and the pulse and symptoms are the signs of deficiency heat of the heart channel. The head-tail method of selecting point, HT 1 (*jí quán*) of the affected channel, is adopted. Reinforcing method of needling is employed.

Summary

Nail-like boil (*Dīng Dú* 疔毒) is characterized by appearing at points on the face, lips, fingers and toes at the beginning and ends of the channels. For example, the ending point of the large intestine channel, LI 20 (*yíng xiāng*), if the boil is here, the starting point, LI 1 (*shāng yáng*), is treated, causing symptoms such as fever, chills, nausea, pain and irritability to quickly disappear after needling. When near the *yuán*-source or *shū*-stream points other points of affected channels may be selected instead of the head-tail points.

If there is lymphatitis, a lancing needle can be used to prick once every inch along the affect area. Or place a slice of ginger at the starting or ending point of a red thread, do moxibustion with cones, till the red thread disappears.

PSORIASIS

Cheng Xin-nong's Medical Record

Yi, 60, first visit was on August 23, 1984

【Chief Complaint】

Tinea with itching at the neck and palms for two years

【Present Medical History】

Two years ago the patient began to have tinea with itching at the palms, afterwards the nape and elbows became involved. The patient was diagnosed with neurodermatitis and treated with various therapies, but the itching was not relieved. He could not sleep at night because of the itching.

【Examination】

The skin of the dorsum of the hands and elbows was rough like cowskin; red tongue, white coating, wiry pulse

【Diagnosis】

Psoriasis (due to wind heat damp retention, disharmony between qi and blood)

【Treatment Principles】

Dispel wind, transform damp, clear heat, moisten dryness

【Treatment】

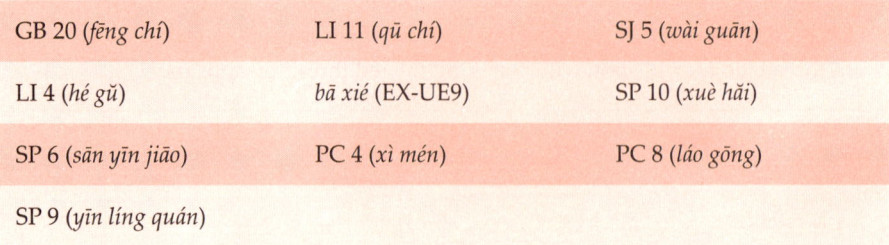

GB 20 (fēng chí)	LI 11 (qū chí)	SJ 5 (wài guān)
LI 4 (hé gǔ)	bā xié (EX-UE9)	SP 10 (xuè hǎi)
SP 6 (sān yīn jiāo)	PC 4 (xì mén)	PC 8 (láo gōng)
SP 9 (yīn líng quán)		

A plum-blossom needle was used to tap the nape, elbow and dorsum of the hands.

Draining method.

【Note】

Due to congenital deficiency and invasion of wind damp heat the channels have become blocked. GB 20 (*fēng chí*) is treated to dispel the wind. LI 11 (*qū chí*) and LI 4 (*hé gǔ*), the *hé*-sea and *yuán* - source of the large intestine channel of the hand *yangming*, clear damp heat in the skin, stop itching, and transform the damp heat. *Bā xié* (EX-UE9) dispels wind, activates channels and stop itching. SJ 5 (*wài guān*) clears heat and removes obstructions from the channels. SP 10 (*xuè hǎi*) nourishes blood to moisten dryness. SP 6 (*sān yīn jiāo*) and SP 9 (*yīn líng quán*) dispel dampness and promote diuresis. "All pain, itching and ulcerations are related to the heart." Drain PC 4 (*xì mén*) and PC 8 (*láo gōng*) to settle the heart, calm the mind, and clear the *ying* - nutritive to stop itching. Using the plum-blossom hammer to treat the nape, elbow and dorsum of hands removes wind toxins from the skin and muscles.

Yang Jie-bin's Medical Record

Qiu, female, 30, first visit was on September 3, 1993

【Chief Complaint】

The nape of her neck and the left elbow had thickened skin with serious itching for three months.

【Present Medical History】

The patient began to have a thickening of the skin with serious itching at the nape and elbow in the past three months. She tried many kinds of treatment, but all to no effect.

【Examination】

The skin of the nape in an area 4 cm × 8 cm and the left cubital fossa in an area 3 cm × 5 cm became thick, dry and chapped, and with serious itching. It was made worse by warmth, and a pink granule-like fluid came out after scratching.

【Diagnosis】

Psoriasis (due to blood deficiency, wind dryness)

【Treatment Principles】

Nourish blood, activate blood, dispel wind, moisten dryness

【Treatment】

The affected areas were tapped with a plum blossom hammer till a little blood leaked out. Cotton moxibustion was applied in this way: A thin layer of cotton was placed on the affected area and ignited. This moxibustion treatment was repeated five times. Treatment was given once every three days.

After one treatment, the itching was greatly relieved. After treatments the itching was almost resolved and the skin in the affected area began to thin. After ten treatments the skin became smooth; nearly normal.

【Note】

According to Professor Yang Jie-bin, in prolonged stubborn tinea diseases, phlegm damp and blood stasis are retained in the channels and collaterals. Causing a *ying* - nutritive and *wei* - defensive imbalance in an already weak constitution. This manifests as blood deficiency and wind dryness. Bleeding is an important aspect of treatment as it removes stasis and allows for new blood production. Cotton moxibustion is also used to improve the curative effect. At the beginning of disease, wind damp heat reside in, and obstruct the flow of qi and blood in the skin. Later there will be blood deficiency and wind dryness, which causes itching and thickening, as the skin is deprived of nourishment. Tapping with the plum blossom hammer regulates and invigorates the blood; cotton moxibustion dispel winds and harmonizes the *ying* - nutritive and *wei* - defensive. In this way, the blood is invigorated and the wind is eliminated, so the itching stops.

246

LEUKODERMA

He Pu-ren's Medical Records

Liu, female,18

【Chief Complaint】
Many white patches all over the body for seven years

【Present Medical History】
Seven years ago, she began to have 1 cm white patches on the lateral side of her left lower limb. One year ago, her wrists, ankles and right hypochondrium began to have white patches too.

【Examination】
The biggest patch was 5 cm × 7 cm. Red tongue with toothmarks on the borders, thin white coating, thready pulse.

【Diagnosis】
Leukoderma (due to disharmony between qi and blood, skin lack of nourishment)

【Treatment Principles】
Regulate qi and blood, nourish skin and muscles

【Treatment】

ā shì (local points)	LU 4 (xiá bái)

The white patches were needled with many short filiform needles and retained for 30 minutes. Moxibustion was done at LU 4 (xiá bái) for 30 minutes.

In total the patient was given 10 treatments, after which the white patches became much smaller, and the one on the left wrist almost disappeared.

【Note】

This patient's skin problem is thought to be caused by qi and blood deficiency, leading to poor nourishment of skin and muscles. The ***Micro-removing method***, (*Wēi Tōng Fǎ* 微通法), in which a filiform needle is used, and the ***Warm-removing method*** (*Wēn Tōng Fǎ* 温通法), in which moxibustion is adopted, are applied to tonify qi and blood, strengthen the normal qi, and dispel pathogenic qi. Moxibustion was done at LU 4 (*xiá bái*) to regulate the qi of the lung. The lung dominates skin and skin hair, it is associated with the white colour, so the appearance of leukoderma is considered to be a disease of the lung. *Plain Questions* says: "All kinds of qi relate to the lung" and "Convergence of the vessels is in the lung". Therefore, moxibustion applied at LU 4 (*xiá bái*) functions to to regulate qi and blood, thus nourishing the skin and muscles.

Fu, female, 27

【Chief Complaint】

White patch on the right shoulder for several months

【Present Medical History】

Several months ago, the patient noticed a white patch on her right shoulder, there was no itchiness or heat. Application of medicine was not effective.

【Examination】

The white patch 3 cm × 2 cm in size, pale tongue, white sticky coating, slippery pulse

【Diagnosis】

Leukoderma (due to damp retention)

【Treatment Principles】

Regulate qi and blood, nourish skin and muscles

【Treatment】

ā shì (local points)

The patch was repeatedly pricked with a thin fire-needle. Treatment was given twice a week. After five treatments the patch disappeared.

【Note】

Looking at the tongue and pulse we see this is a damp retention presentation, which leads to disharmony of the qi and blood failing to nourish the skin and muscles. As the damp is a yin pathogenic factor, fire needling promotes yang and removes obstructions from the channels. This treatment strengthens the normal qi that then drives the pathogenic damp from the channels and collaterals.

Sun, male, 30

【Chief Complaint】

White patch on the dorsum of the left hand for half a month

【Present Medical History】

Half a month ago the patient noticed a white patch on the dorsum of his left hand after a quarrel with somebody.

【Examination】

The white patch 3 cm × 6 cm in size, red tongue, thin white coating, rolling pulse

【Diagnosis】

Leukoderma (due to qi stagnation, blood stasis)

【Treatment Principles】

Regulate qi and blood, nourish skin and muscles

【Treatment】

ā shì (local points)

Once a week the white patch was bled and cupped. After four treatments the patch disappeared.

【Note】

His patch is thought to be related with anger, which damages the liver, causing qi stagnation. "*Qi* is the commander of blood, blood is the mother of qi." Qi stagnation leads to blood stasis, thus skin and muscles lack nourishment, resulting in leukoderma. Bleeding, which is considered a *Strong-removing method*, (*Qiáng Tōng Fǎ* 强通法), directly removes blood stasis. When the channels are unobstructed the qi and blood circulate well to nourish skin and muscles.

Summary

Leukoderma, called *Bái Bó Fēng* (白驳风), is a localized pigmentation disease. It is due to hereditary, autoimmune and nervous factors. In TCM, it can be due to emotional disturbance, qi stagnation, invasion of exogenous pathogenic factors, the failure of lung defensive qi, or qi and blood disharmony giving rise to poor nourishment of the skin. Professor He Pu-ren says that skin patches are only the outward manifestation of the disease, the root of the disease is a disharmony of the qi and blood. Treatment principles are to nourish blood, dispel wind, regulate qi and blood to nourish the skin.

Three-removing method (*Sān Tōng Fǎ* 三通法); different needles are used according to the individual condition of patients.

For those with qi and blood deficiency, the Micro-removing method (*Wēi Tōng Fǎ*), with the filiform needle, used together with Warm-removing method (*Wēn Tōng Fǎ* 温通法) (moxibustion) nourishes qi and blood to strengthen the normal qi. When strong the normal qi will overcome the pathogenic qi.

For those with damp retention, the Warm-removing method with the fire needling to tonify yang to transform damp is used to warm the channels and collaterals and move qi to invigorate the blood.

For those with qi stagnation and blood stasis the Strong-removing method (*Qiáng Tōng Fǎ*) of bleeding to dredge the channels and collaterals is applied to remove stasis directly.

Yĭn Zhĕn (URTICARIA)

Record in *Acupuncture - Moxibustion for Difficult Diseases* (*Qí Nán Zá Bìng Zhēn Jiŭ Zhì Liáo*)

Zhou, female, 34, first visit was on June 10, 1999

【Chief Complaint】
Itchy skin for one year

【Present Medical History】
Scattered skin rashes with itching, irritability, thirst, and yellow urine. Anti-histamines did not help.

【Examination】
Slightly raised, itchy, patchy red. Red tongue, slight yellow coating, superficial and wiry pulse.

【Diagnosis】
Urticaria (*Yĭn Zhĕn*) (due to wind heat attacking body surface)

【Treatment Principles】
Dispel wind, harmonize the ying

【Treatment】

SP 10 (*xuè hăi*)	LI 11 (*qū chí*)	GB 31 (*fēng shì*)
SP 6 (*sān yīn jiāo*)	DU 14 (*dà zhuī*)	

Treatment was given once a day, 12 times as one course. After two courses she was cured.

【Note】
SP 10 (*xuè hăi*) clears the blood heat. LI 11 (*qū chí*) functions to clear

wind heat, remove rashes and stop itching. GB 31 (*fēng shì*) "wind city" is needled to dispel wind. SP 6 (*sān yīn jiāo*) nourishes qi and blood. DU 14 (*dà zhuī*) an intersecting point of the yang channels drives out wind heat.

Summary

Yǐn Zhěn (hidden rash 瘾疹), also called *Fēng Zhěn* (wind rash 风疹), is urticaria in modern medicine. It is an allergic skin disease induced by multiple pathogenic factors, with symptoms of itching, skin rashes, and wheals that come and go, and do not leave any permanent mark.

Main points: LI 11 (*qū chí*), LI 4 (*hé gǔ*), SP 10 (*xuè hǎi*), and GB 20 (*fēng chí*).

Bleed BL 17 (*gé shù*) and PC 3 (*qū zé*) for those with rashes that are red in colour. Add ST 36 (*zú sān lǐ*) for those with white coloured rashes. Add PC 6 (*nèi guān*) and RN 12 (*zhōng wǎn*) for those with epigastric pain.

ACNE

Feng Li's Medical Record

Gao, female, 30

【**Chief Complaint**】
Acne on the face with repeated attacks for six months

【**Present Medical History**】
This patient had severe outbreaks of pustulating acne whenever she ate deep-fried food, seafood or drank alcohol, along with a dry mouth and bad breath, and constipation.

【**Examination**】
Red tongue, yellow greasy coating, slippery rapid pulse

【Diagnosis】

Acne (due to accumulated heat in the lung and stomach)

【Treatment Principles】

Promote the lung in dispersing, clear heat, transform damp

【Treatment】

DU 14 (dà zhuī)	BL 13 (fèi shù)	BL 15 (xīn shù)
BL 17 (gé shù)	BL 21 (wèi shù)	BL 25 (dà cháng shù)

A three-edged needle was used to bleed 3~4 points, which were then cupped for 5 minutes to draw out more blood. The patient was treated once a day, 10 times as one course.

Auricular points: lung, large intestine, endocrine, adrenal, cheek, and forehead.

Herbal seeds were applied to ear points. Ears were alternately treated. The points were stimulated by the patient three times a day, 10 days as one course of treatment. After the first course of treatment her acne was reduced, and her stools improved. After three courses all the acne disappeared.

【Note】

This is a syndrome of accumulated heat in the lung and stomach with heat toxins attacking upward. Bleeding DU 14 (dà zhuī) clears heat toxins and disperses pathogenic factors from the skin and muscles. BL 13 (fèi shù) and BL 21 (wèi shù) clear heat from the lung and stomach. Bleeding BL 17 (gé shù), the influential point of blood, invigorates the blood and removes heat toxins. BL 25 (dà cháng shù) dredges the large intestine and treats constipation. After lancing with a three-edged needle, cupping is applied to increase the stasis removing effect and to drive out the pathogenic heat; this is the meaning of "stasis should be driven out." Acne is always accompanied by hyperactive *yangming* fire. The lung and large intestine are externally internally related. The auricle point for the large intestine is selected to clear *yangming* fire. "All kinds of pain, itching and boils are related to the heart", so the heart is also treated to clear fire and stop itching. The endocrine and adrenal points are used to regulate the endocrine system. The cheek and forehead points are corresponding points for acne on face, thus are treated to improve blood circulation to the facial region. And deep-fried and spicy food should be avoided, and more fruits and vegetables should be eaten to prevent constipation. Facial hygiene and physical exercises are self care measures the patient should undertake on their own.

Summary

Acne is a chronic inflammatory skin disease of the hair follicles and sebaceous glands. It is mostly seen in the facial region of teenagers and middle aged females, and can seriously affect their appearance. TCM holds that overindulging in rich foods damages the spleen and stomach, which then produces damp heat that steams upward. Or, it can be caused from accumulated heat in the lung or invasion of wind.

Accumulated heat in lung: in the early stage there is redness, swelling, pain, itching, dry mouth, yellow urine, dry stools, a red tongue with a yellow coating, and a floating and rapid pulse.

Damp heat in the spleen and stomach: the acne comes and goes, yellow greasy fluid or pus can be squeezed out, the face is oily, there is bad breath and a bitter taste in the mouth, occassionally a poor appetite, sticky stools or incomplete stools, red tongue with a yellow greasy coating, and a wiry rapid pulse.

Qi and blood stagnation: dark, purple acne that is chronic in nature, accompanied by papillae, pustules, nodules, and cysts.

Prescription I: Main points: LI 4 (*hé gǔ*), GB 20 (*fēng chí*).

Local points: SI 18 (*quán liáo*), ST 7 (*xià guān*), LI 20 (*yíng xiāng*), and ST 2 (*sì bái*).

Add BL 13 (*fèi shù*) and LU 7 (*liè quē*) for wind heat in the lung; LI 11 (*qū chí*), ST 40 (*fēng lóng*), SP 9 (*yīn líng quán*) and SP 6 (*sān yīn jiāo*) for damp heat of the spleen and stomach; SP 10 (*xuè hǎi*), SP 6 (*sān yīn jiāo*) and LV 3 (*tài chōng*) for qi and blood stagnation; and SJ 6 (*zhī gōu*), SP 15 (*dà héng*), KI 6 (*zhào hǎi*) and SP 6 (*sān yīn jiāo*) for constipation.

Prescription II: DU 14 (*dà zhuī*), BL 20 (*pí shù*), ST 36 (*zú sān lǐ*), LI 4 (*hé gǔ*), and SP 6 (*sān yīn jiāo*).

Ear points: lung, shenmen, sympathetic nerve, endocrine, adrenal, subcortex.

Manipulation: Stick vaccaria seeds (*Wáng Bù Liú Xíng Zǐ*) with adhesive plaster to the ear points. Press the points three times a day, 10 minutes each time.

CHLOASMA

Feng Li's Medical Record

Zhang, female, 42

【Chief Complaint】

Abnormal facial pigmentation for one year

【Present Medical History】

One year ago, she began to experience abnormal facial pigmentation that gradually became darker; accompanied with listlessness, insomnia, scanty light colored menstrual flow.

【Examination】

Pale tongue, white coating, thready pulse

【Diagnosis】

Chloasma (qi and blood deficiency)

【Treatment Principles】

Regulate the *zang-fu*, replenish qi and blood, remove pigmentation, improve her appearance

【Treatment】

Pigmentation area		LI 4 (*hé gǔ*)		SP 6 (*sān yīn jiāo*)	
ST 36 (*zú sān lǐ*)		BL 20 (*pí shù*)		BL 23 (*shèn shù*)	
BL 18 (*gān shù*)					
Ear points:	Cheek	lung	liver	spleen	Kidney
Endocrine	Shenmen	Ovary	Internal genitalia		Uterus

The body points were treated and needles retained for 30 minutes after the arrival of qi. Treatment was given once a day, 10 times as one course. The ear points were stimulated with vaccaria seeds, two ears alternately treated.

After the first course of treatment the pigmentation became lighter and the accompanying symptoms reduced. After five courses the chloasma disappeared. The follow-up for one year found no recurrence.

【Note】

In this case the pigmentation is due to qi and blood deficiency, leading to a lack of nourishment of the skin on the face. Needling the local area regulates qi, activates blood, and improves nourishment to the face, which improves cell regeneration and removes accumulated waste, thus reducing the abnormal pigmentation.

LI 4 (*hé gǔ*) is for all diseases of the facial region. SP 6 (*sān yīn jiāo*) regulates the qi of the liver, spleen and kidney. ST 36 (*zú sān lǐ*) strengthens the spleen and stomach, tonifying the post-heaven foundation of the body. BL 18 (*gān shù*), BL 20 (*pí shù*) and BL 23 (*shèn shù*) promote the spleen, liver and kidney function.

Choice of ear points for chloasma follow the theory of ear- *zang-fu* - channels relationship: "The ear is the convergence of all channels", and "*Qi* and blood of 12 channels and 365 collaterals go up to the face and ear. Hearing is formed with the qi of the divergent channels going to the ear." Stimulation of those points relating to chloasma removes obstructions from the channels, regulates qi and blood, transforms stasis, and tonifies the liver and kidney.

Summary

Chloasma is a change in the colour of the face. It mostly appears on the cheek and forehead before and after giving birth.

Prescription I: BL 13 (*fèi shù*), BL 18 (*gān shù*), BL 20 (*pí shù*), BL 19 (*dǎn shù*), BL 23 (*shèn shù*), BL 22 (*sān jiāo shù*), SP 10 (*xuè hǎi*), KI 3 (*tài xī*), and LV 3 (*tài chōng*).

Cupping is on the the Back-*shù* points after needling.

Prescription II: DU 14 (*dà zhuī*), BL 13 (*fèi shù*), BL 17 (*gé shù*), BL 15 (*xīn shù*), and BL 18 (*gān shù*).

Use one point each time, bleed or tap with a plum blossom hammer until the skin turns red, then cup. The points are used by turns, once a day for strong patients and once every 2~3 days for weak ones. Five times as one course, with 3~5 days of rest before the next course.

Ear points: Main points: endocrine, ovary, cheek.

Added points: subcortex, lung, liver, spleen, heart, kidney, adrenal, internal genitalia, eye, mouth, forehead, temple.

Select points according to the affected *zang-fu* and channels and location of brown spots. Endocrine, subcortex and internal genitalia are used in turn.

Manipulation: Stick vaccaria seeds (*Wáng Bù Liú Xíng Zǐ*) with adhesive plaster to the ear points. The patient is asked to press them 3 times a day, 10 minutes each time. Change seeds once every 3~4 days in summer, and 5~6 days in other seasons. Two ears are used alternately.

SPRAIN AND CONTUSION

Yang Jie-bin's Medical Record

Xu, female, 16 years old

【Chief Complaint】

Swelling and pain of the right ankle joint for one day

【Present Medical History】

This patient sprained her right ankle, the joint swelled up and turned black and blue; it was extremely painful. She could not walk at all and could not sleep either because of the pain.

【Examination】

Severely swollen right ankle, unable to put any weight on it at all. There were no fractures or dislocated bones. Pale red tongue, thin white coating, superficial tight pulse.

【Diagnosis】

Sprain

【Treatment Principles】

Activate blood, transform stasis, relieve swelling, stop pain

【Treatment】

GB 40 (*qiū xū*)	BL 60 (*kūn lún*)	ST 41 (*jiě xī*)
ā shì (local points)		

Ā shì points on the affected were bled and cupped. After treatment, the pain was greatly relieved. On the following day the same treatment was given, after which the swelling basically disappeared. After the third session, her swelling and pain stopped completely and she could walk freely.

【Note】

The swelling and pain of the ankle joint is from the blood stasis and qi stagnation. In TCM it is considered *Shāng Jīn* (injury of tendons); in modern medicine it is a soft tissue injury. *Plain Questions - On the Corresponding Relationship Between* Yin *and* Yang *of Man and All Things and That of Seasons (Sù Wèn: Yīn Yáng Yìng Xiàng Dà Lùn*, 素问 • 阴阳应象大论) says: "*Qi* is injured, causing pain, tissue is injured, causing swelling." So the manifestation is swelling and pain. The treatment principle is to move the blood, remove the obstruction of channels, relieve swelling and stop pain. Points of the affected channels in the local area are selected as the main ones to be bled and cupped to "remove blood stasis from the channels to restore the balance of yin and yang."

Summary

Sprain and *contusion* refers here to the injury of soft tissues, including the skin, muscles, tendons, and dislocations caused by violent movement, falls, or overtwisting resulting in local stagnation of qi and blood in the channels of the affected areas that manifests with pain and swelling of the injured areas and motor impairment of the joints. For the treatment, *ā shì* (local points) are used in combination with distal points of the involved channels; this activates blood circulation. Bleeding and cupping of the local area, and application of moxibustion not only relieve swelling and pain, but also speed up the recovery of the injured tissues.

GANGLION

Yang Yong-xuan's Medical Record

Sun, female, 56

【Chief Complaint】

A cyst on the dorsum of her right wrist for several months

【Present Medical History】

The cyst was as big as a longan fruit, movable, and painful when pressed

【Diagnosis】

Ganglion

【Treatment Principles】

Remove stagnation, warm and unobstruct the channels

【Treatment】

In the cyst area, Triple Puncture (*Qī Cì* Needling) was applied. This is a technique in which the needles are inserted at three spots simultaneously; one in the centre of the cyst and two on either side. Warming needle moxibustion was also applied.

The cyst gradually became softer and smaller, and cured after four treatments.

【Note】

Ganglion, called *Jīn Jié* (tendon knot) in TCM, is a hard cyst often occurring at on the wrist or ankle. It is caused by fatigue damaging the tendons.

Summary

For the treatment of *ganglions*, the jelly-like fluid should be drained out with one of the following methods:

a. Use a thick acupuncture needle, prick to break the ganglion from its top, squeeze the jelly fluid out. One week later, repeat the procedure if the cyst reappears.

b. Warming needle method. For mild cases insert one needle deeply into the center of ganglion, then warm with moxa on the needle. After several treatments the ganglion should disappear. For chronic cases use the Triple Puncture (*Qī Cì* Needling); the needles are inserted at three spots with one in the centre and two on either side.

c. Surround with filiform needles. Insert two needles at the base of ganglion, making a "+" inside it, then insert one needle from the top. After removing the needles, press to force out the jelly fluid.

d. Fire needling. Push the ganglion away to one side, heat the needle on an alcohol burner until it is red hot, pierce the ganglion deeply, avoiding any blood vessels, then squeeze out the jelly fluid.

CHAPTER 5 OTHERS

Internal Diseases

Gynecological and Pediatric Diseases

Diseases of Eyes, Ears, Nose and Throat

Skin Diseases, External Diseases

Others

SUN STROKE

Yang Jie-bin's Medical Record

Xia, female, 29

【Chief Complaint】

Headache and nausea for two hours

【Present Medical History】

The patient had a splitting headache, with irritability, strong thirst, profuse sweating, and nausea.

【Examination】

Sickly complexion, rough breathing, red eyes. T: 41℃(106℉). Yellow slippery coating, soft rapid pulse

【Diagnosis】

Sunstroke (summer-heat damaging the mind)

【Treatment Principles】

Open the orifices, reduce body temperature, dispel summer heat

【Treatment】

DU 14 (dà zhuī)	tài yáng (EX-HN5)	LI 1 (shāng yáng)
PC 9 (zhōng chōng)	SI 1 (shào zé)	BL 40 (wěi zhōng)

DU 14 (dà zhuī) was bled and cupped. Other points were bled without cupping. She was given warm light saline to drink.

Two hours later, her fever was reduced and her mind was again clear. She went home by herself.

【Note】

Serious cases of sunstroke may manifest with loss of consciousness, profuse sweating, cold extremities, shallow and abrupt respiration, and a feeble pulse. For the treatment, Professor Yang Jie-bin's Five-Center points DU 20 (*bǎi huì*) along with PC 8 (*láo gōng*) and KI 1 (*yǒng quán*) is recommended. The effect is better and with faster results if acupuncture and moxibustion are used together to stimulate DU 26 (*rén zhōng*) and *shí xuān* (EX-UE11).

Summary

Sunstroke is an acute condition in which the body's thermo-regulatory function becomes disordered due to exposure to scorchingly hot summer sun; it can also be accompanied by peripheral circulatory failure. There are accompanying symptoms of dizziness, headache, and nausea; in severe cases there can be convulsions or sudden loss of consciousness. Professor Yang Jie-bin treats this with good clinical results by bleeding. From his many years clinical practice, he has summarized two groups of points called Clearing Summer-heat Prescription.

a. DU 14 (*dà zhuī*), *tài yáng* (EX-HN5), LI 1 (*shāng yáng*), PC 9 (*zhōng chōng*), SI 1 (*shào zé*), and BL 40 (*wěi zhōng*).

b. BL 11 (*dà zhù*), BL 2 (*cuán zhú*), LU 11 (*shào shāng*), SJ 1 (*guān chōng*), *shí xuān* (EX-UE11), and PC 3 (*qū zé*).

Usage: Bleed and cup DU 14 (*dà zhuī*) and BL 11 (*dà zhù*), draw out 4~5 ml of dark blood. Bleed 0.5~1 ml from the other points. PC 3 (*qū zé*) and BL 40 (*wěi zhōng*) can bleed 3~4 ml.

Explanation: The extreme hot weather in summer causes sunstroke in those with a weak constitution. DU 14 (*dà zhuī*) and BL 11 (*dà zhù*) are selected to clear heat through bleeding. *Tài yáng* (EX-HN5) and BL 2 (*cuán zhú*) clear heat of the upper *jiao*. Summer heat is a yang pathogenic factor, it is likely to affect the pericardium, and damage the qi and yin of the human body. PC 3 (*qū zé*) and BL 40 (*wěi zhōng*) clear heat from the pericardium and blood. The *jǐng*-well points and *shí xuān* (EX-UE11), the meeting places of yin and yang channels, are needled to clear heat from the qi and yin and open the orifices.

If the summer heat affects the pericardium, misting the heart and manifests as loss of consciousness, DU 26 (*rén zhōng*) and DU 20 (*bǎi huì*) are treated to promote resuscitation. For restlessness, add PC 6 (*nèi guān*) and HT 7 (*shén mén*) to settle the heart and calm the mind. For convulsions, add SI 3 (*hòu xī*), GB 34 (*yáng líng quán*) and BL 57 (*chéng shān*) to relax the muscles. For vomiting and diarrhea, add RN 12 (*zhōng wǎn*), ST 25 (*tiān shū*) and ST 36 (*zú sān lǐ*) to harmonize the middle *jiao* and regulate the *fu*-intestine qi. For dizziness and blurred vision, add *sì shén cōng* (EX-HN1) and LV 3 (*tài chōng*) to remove wind yang. For sweating, cold limbs and a hidden pulse, apply a significant amount of moxibustion at RN 4 (*guān yuán*), RN 6 (*qì hǎi*) and DU 20 (*bǎi huì*) to restore yang to treat collapse.

OBESITY

Tan Xiao-hong's Medical Record

X X, female, 53, first visit was on January 8, 1995

【Chief Complaint】
Obesity for 12 years

【Present Medical History】
She had a history of obesity for 12 years, now her body weight is about 300 pounds. She had a voracious appetite and shortness of breath on exertion.

【Examination】
Yellow and slightly greasy coating, slippery pulse

【Diagnosis】
Obesity (due to phlegm damp retention)

【Treatment Principles】
Transform phlegm damp, regulate qi of the middle *jiao*

【Treatment】

ST 34 (*liáng qiū*)	SP 4 (*gōng sūn*)	PC 6 (*nèi guān*)

ST 40 (*fēng lóng*)	ST 36 (*zú sān lǐ*)			
Ear points:	lung	Endocrine	*Sanjiao*	stomach
	Intestine	Shenmen	Hunger	

A draining method was used for the body points. Treatment was given twice a week. Ear points were stimulated with vaccaria seeds, which were changed once every three days. The two ears were used alternately.

She was asked to press the ear points several times before meals, eat more vegetables, less oily food, and get more exercise. After the treatments in the first week she felt good. She said that pressing the ear points reduced her appetite and she lost four pounds; she felt confident. After more than 20 treatments she had lost 42 pounds. The palpitations and shortness of breath disappeared. She was in a good mood.

【Note】

Obesity, according to TCM, it is due to phlegm. "Fat people have phlegm and slim people have fire." Long term phlegm retention transforms into heat. Heat in the stomach will cause people to feel hungry all the time. Treating this problem mostly involves the use of points from the spleen and stomach channels. ST 40 (*fēng lóng*) and ST 36 (*zú sān lǐ*) function to strengthen the spleen and transform phlegm. ST 34 (*liáng qiū*), the *xī*-cleft point of the foot *yangming* stomach channel and SP 4 (*gōng sūn*), the *luò*-connecting point of the foot *taiyin* spleen channel, regulate the spleen and stomach, transform phlegm, and reduce stomach heat. PC 6 (*nèi guān*) regulates stomach qi. Modern medicine reports that puncturing SP 4 (*gōng sūn*), PC 6 (*nèi guān*) and ST 34 (*liáng qiū*) functions to inhibit gastric acid secretion and needling SP 4 (*gōng sūn*) weakens gastric peristalsis. The ear points: lung, *sanjiao*, spleen and stomach function to regulate absorption and excretion, promote metabolism and induce diuresis. The endocrine point regulates the endocrine system. Using a combination of body and ear points, the metabolism of the human body can be regulated and the appetite can be reduced leading to a decrease in body weight.

Summary

Points to treat obesity

Main points: RN 12 (*zhōng wǎn*), RN 9 (*shuǐ fēn*), RN 4 (*guān yuán*), SP 6 (*sān yīn jiāo*), ST 26 (*wài líng*), ST 25 (*tiān shū*), and ST 24 (*huá ròu mén*).

Supplementary points: LI 11 (*qū chí*), LI 4 (*hé gǔ*), ST 37 (*shàng jù xū*), and ST 44 (*nèi tíng*) for excess heat of the stomach and intestines. Treat ST 36 (*zú sān lǐ*), ST 40 (*fēng lóng*), and SP 9 (*yīn líng quán*) for phlegm damp retention. To tonify spleen and kidney qi needle ST 36 (*zú sān lǐ*), SP 6 (*sān yīn jiāo*), BL 20 (*pí shù*), BL 23 (*shèn shù*). Needle SJ 6 (*zhī gōu*) through to PC 6 (*nèi guān*), and add ST 36 (*zú sān lǐ*), ST 37 (*shàng jù xū*) for constipation. LI 11 (*qū chí*) and LV 3 (*tài chōng*) are used for hypertension. To treat coronary heart disease PC 6 (*nèi guān*), SP 6 (*sān yīn jiāo*), and RN 17 (*dàn zhōng*) are the points to select. Should there be diabetes, add ST 36 (*zú sān lǐ*), SP 6 (*sān yīn jiāo*), and SJ 4 (*yáng chí*). To reduce abdominal fat above umbilicus select RN 13 (*shàng wǎn*), ST 22 (*guān mén*), or ST 24 (*huá ròu mén*). SP 14 (*fù jié*), ST 27 (*dà jù*), ST 28 (*shuǐ dào*) are used for reducing abdominal fat below the umbilicus. GB 26 (*dài mài*), GB 31 (*fēng shì*), BL 52 (*zhì shì*) can be used to slim the waist region. BL 54 (*zhì biān*), BL 36 (*chéng fú*), and *ā shì* (local points) reduce fat around the hips. For fatty upper limbs, needle LI 14 (*bì nào*), LI 15 (*jiān yú*), LI 11 (*qū chí*); use ST 32 (*fú tù*), ST 34 (*liáng qiū*), ST 40 (*fēng lóng*), *ā shì* (local points) for reducing fat of the lower limbs.

Generally, 2~3 inch filiform needles are used, needle using a draining or even method, once everyday or every other day, 30~60 minutes with retention of the needles. Fifteen treatments constitutes one course with three days of rest before the next course.

Ear points: Endocrine, brain point, stomach, spleen, kidney, liver, large intestine, lung, heart.

Five or six points are selected each time, treatment is given once or twice a week. The ears are alternately treated; with the patient stimulating before meals everyday.

In addition to treatment attention must be paid to the diet, life style and exercises. Especially, after weight has been lost, emphasis on lifestyle habits is critical.

CHRONIC FATIGUE SYNDROME

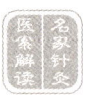 ## He Pu-ren's Medical Record

X X, male, 41, first visit was on September 6, 2004

【Chief Complaint】

Insomnia for two weeks, headache for one week

【Present Medical History】

This patient was a policeman, due to work pressure he began to have insomnia two weeks ago; after that he had headaches, was fatigued, had a short fuse and was irritable.

【Examination】

BP: 140/80 mm Hg. Tip and borders of tongue red, coating yellow sticky and slightly dry, pulse wiry and slippery.

【Diagnosis】

Chronic fatigue syndrome (due to liver yang hyperactivity)

【Treatment】

BL 43 (gāo huāng)	BL 17 (gé shù)	BL 19 (dǎn shù)

Strong-removing method (Qiáng Tōng Fǎ) was adopted in that the points were lanced, bled and then cupped to promote an even greater discharge of blood. More blood, more effect. The patient was treated once a week. Generally, after 1~3 treatments satisfactory results will be achieved.

After one treatment, the patient felt better and his sleep improved. After three treatments his insomnia disappeared. He was cured later with herbal medication.

【Note】

BL 43 (gāo huāng) is located below the spinous process of the 4th thoracic vertebra and 3 inches lateral to the midline; BL 17 (gé shù) is located below the spinous process of the 7th thoracic vertebra and 1.5 inches lateral to the midline, and BL 19 (dǎn shù) is located below the spinous process of the 10th thoracic vertebra and 1.5 inches lateral to the midline, the latter two are known as the *Four-Flower Points*. The ancient acupuncture literature reports that these points are used to treat the chronic deficiency diseases that are similar to today's chronic illnesses. Many clinical reports and lab experiments have shown these points to be extremely effective for deficiency diseases.

Strong-removing method (*Qiáng Tōng Fǎ* 强通法) — *One of the He's Three removing methods is (Sān Tōng Fǎ* 三通法*). It is a techique that focuses regulating the blood by bleeding the superficial veins at certain areas of the body; this regulates the qi and blood of the zang-fu organs.*

Summary

Chronic fatigue syndrome (CFS), is a chronic illness where the body is in a long term subacute state of health that is characterized by a low quality of life as there are numerous manifestations of somatic and psychological symptoms. The somatic symptoms include profound fatigue, accompanied by sleep disturbances, headache, lowered resistance and metabolism disorders. The psychological symptoms include anxiety, depression, irritability, restlessness, hot temper, and constant feeling of fear.

Prescription I: BL 43 (*gāo huāng*), Four-Flower points. He's Strong-Removing method (*Qiáng Tōng Fǎ*).

Prescription II: Main points: BL 15 (*xīn shù*), BL 18 (*gān shù*), BL 20 (*pí shù*), BL 23 (*shèn shù*), and BL 13 (*fèi shù*).

Supplementary points: ST 36 (*zú sān lǐ*) and DU 20 (*bǎi huì*) for qi deficiency. RN 4 (*guān yuán*) and RN 6 (*qì hǎi*) for qi and blood deficiency. SP 6 (*sān yīn jiāo*) and RN 6 (*qì hǎi*) for qi and yin deficiency; LV 3 (*tài chōng*) and ST 36 (*zú sān lǐ*) for qi deficiency and liver qi stagnation. ST 36 (*zú sān lǐ*) and SP 6 (*sān yīn jiāo*) for qi deficiency with blood stasis. LV 3 (*tài chōng*) and SP 9 (*yīn líng quán*) for disharmony between the liver and spleen. DU 4 (*mìng mén*) and BL 25 (*dà cháng shù*) for spleen and kidney yang deficiency. KI 3 (*tài xī*) and LV 3 (*tài chōng*) for liver and kidney yin deficiency.

The Back-*shù* points are the sites where the qi of the *zang-fu* organs gathers. Needling the Back-*shù* points regulates the qi of the *zang-fu* organs. With normal circulation of qi and blood, all the tissues and organs of the human body are well nourished and will not feel fatigued.

ABSTINENCE SYNDROME

Tan Xiao-hong's Medical Record

X X, female, 63, first visit was on February 18, 1995

【Chief Complaint】
Smoking cigarettes for 35 years

【Present Medical History】
This patient smoked more than 35 cigarettes everyday. She tried many times to stop smoking but failed. It happened she heard that acupuncture could help stop smoking, so she came to try.

【Diagnosis】
Smoking withdrawal syndrome

【Treatment】

tián měi (EX-UE) for stopping smoking

She was asked to inhale and hold her breath when the needle was inserted and after insertion to exhale. The needle was rotated. Ten minutes later, she tried to smoke and felt tasteless and had no desire to finish this cigarette. The needle was removed after retaining for 20 minutes.

Ear points:	Mouth	*Lung*	*Sanjiao*	Endocrine

Herbal vaccaria seeds were stuck at the ear points and the patient pressed them several times a day. On the 4th day she came in and said that she stopped smoking completely, the only problem was that she felt like she had lost something and did not known what to do with both hands. The same treatment was given and she was told not to worry. One week later she felt normal and she was in a good mood. She was still smoke free when she came in for a one month follow up visit.

【Note】

Tián měi (EX-UE) is a specific point to stop smoking that was accidentally discovered by the American doctor James. S. Olms. *Tián měi* means after giving up cigarettes the patient can taste the deliciousness of food. Its location is generally described at the midpoint between LI 5 (*yáng xī*) and LU 7 (*liè quē*). But treatment given here is not very effective. According to Dr. James. S. Olms, it is at about one finger-breadth from the border of the styloid process of the radius, in the small soft depression near LU 7 (*liè quē*). Olms thinks that most practitioners have problems finding the depression by palpation, but if you use a curved nose forceps to press around LU 7 (*liè quē*), it is easy to find. The needle can be inserted 3~4mm into the depression without falling over, like a key into a lock. If the point is not precisely located, if you are even off by 1~2mm, the needle will not stand up, and the result will not be as good as it could be. *Tián měi* (EX-UE) is a good point to help people stop smoking, the important thing is to be sure it is precisely located.

Fan Hong's Medical Record

Wang, female, 25

【Chief Complaint】

Addiction to heroin for seven years

【Present Medical History】

Seven years ago, she began to smoke heroin because she was curious about it. Gradually she smoked as much as 3g five or six times a day. She would pass out, and then three hours later wake up and smoke again. All day long she was in a half anaesthetized state. When she did not smoke she would have withdrawal symptoms and so continued to smoke to avoid them. She tried quitting seven times, but failed each time. When she came in for drug rehabilitation, it was 30 hours after her use of heroin.

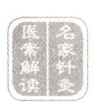

【Examination】

Clear consciousness, listlessness, pupils 0. 25cm, symmetrical, sensitive light reflex, heart rate 96/min, regular rhythm, body weight 47kg, skin looking like chicken skin, frequent yawning, excessive tearing, nausea, vomiting, irritability with sensations like a cat scratching her heart and ants walking in her bones.

【Diagnosis】

Heroin withdrawal syndrome

【Treatment】

DU 14 (*dà zhuī*)	HT 7 (*shén mén*)	PC 6 (*nèi guān*)

shí xuān (EX-UE11)

The needle was rotated continuously for 5 minutes with strong stimulation. S*hí xuān* (EX-UE11) was bled. DU 14 (*dà zhuī*) and PC 6 (*nèi guān*) were used alternately each time. Additional points were selected accordingly.

On the following day, her nausea, vomiting, running nose and tears were obviously less, and sleep was better. Now she felt soreness and fatigue in the low back, and her chicken skin was much relieved. LI 1 (*shāng yáng*) and GB 41 (*zú lín qì*) were added for treatment.

On the third day, the withdrawal symptoms basically stopped. She slept very lightly and found it difficult to fall a sleep again. There was not any more chicken skin. KI 1 (*yǒng quán*) and DU 20 (*bǎi huì*) were added.

On the fourth day, her sleep was not good. She had soreness in the low back. Her pupils, heart rate, blood pressure and skin were normal.

On the seventh day, her urine test was clean. Her withdrawal symptoms disappeared. The body weight increased to 49kg.

【Note】

The main points are PC 6 (*nèi guān*) and DU 14 (*dà zhuī*). Each time use one of them. On the first day HT 9 (*shào chōng*) and HT 7 (*shén mén*) were added. On the second day LI 1 (*shāng yáng*) and GB 41 (*zú lín qì*) added. On the third day LI 4 (*hé gǔ*) and ST 36 (*zú sān lǐ*) or SP 4 (*gōng sūn*) and SJ 6 (*zhī gōu*) were added to treat gastrointestinal tract symptoms. HT 7 (*shén mén*) and SP 6 (*sān yīn jiāo*) or DU 20 (*bǎi huì*) and KI 1 (*yǒng quán*) added to deal with her insomnia. DU 26 (*shuǐ gōu*) and KI 1 (*yǒng quán*) were treated to settle her will. PC 9 (*zhōng chōng*) and PC 8 (*láo gōng*) or *shí xuān* (EX-UE11) and DU 14 (*dà zhuī*) were added for serious irritability.

PC 6 (*nèi guān*) sedates the heart and calms the mind, regulates qi in the chest, harmonizes the stomach to stop vomiting. DU 14 (*dà zhuī*) ascends yang and nourishes qi, removes heat and tonifies deficiency. HT 9 (*shào chōng*) opens the orifices, clears the mind and reduces toxic heat. HT 7 (*shén mén*) calms the mind and clears fire from the *Ying*-nutritive. LI 1 (*shāng yáng*) opens the orifices, clears heat and stops spasm. GB 41 (*zú lín qì*) dispels wind, reduces fire and clears the mind. LI 4 (*hé gǔ*) harmonizes the stomach and removes obstruction of the intestines. ST 36 (*zú sān lǐ*) regulates the intestines and stomach and reinforces the normal qi. SP 4 (*gōng sūn*) the *luò*-connecting point, which also opens the *chong* vessel, regulates the spleen and stomach. SJ 6 (*zhī gōu*) clears heat and promotes bowel movements. SP 6 (*sān yīn jiāo*), the intersecting point of the three foot yin channels, especially strengthens the spleen and calms the mind. DU 20 (*bǎi huì*), known as Three-*Yang* Five-*Hui* (*Sān Yáng Wǔ Huì*), is especially effective in calming the mind and soothing the liver. DU 26 (*shuǐ gōu*), KI 1 (*yǒng quán*), PC 9 (*zhōng chōng*), PC 8 (*láo gōng*) and *shí xuān* (EX-UE11) open the orifices and clear heart fire.

The above-mentioned points activate channel qi, tonify normal qi, remove pathogenic qi, regulate yin and yang, and simultaneously treat both the branch (*Biāo* 标) and root (*Běn* 本) of drug-addiction.

This case report comes from the Shanghai Police Bureau Rehabilitation Center. In the report PC 6 (nèi guān) and DU 14 (dà zhuī) are used as the main points for the treatment of 20 cases of heroin withdrawal. During the treatment process no opiates or sedatives of any kind were allowed to be taken. The result was that 19 of the addicts made it through the withdrawal process, indicating that acupuncture can help relieve the symptoms of heroin withdrawal.

Ci Shui-xin and Shang Yin-jia's Medical Record

X X, male, 27, first visit was on November 14, 1993

【Chief Complaint】

Heroin smoking for six years

【Present Medical History】

Everyday this patient smoked about 1g two to three times a day. In the past two years, being aware of its harmfulness, he tried to quit, but failed twice. Now he came for acupuncture treatment. He had dizziness with blurred vision and weakness throughout the whole body. Additionally he had nasal congestion, poor appetite, insomnia, forgetfulness, and at night he could fall asleep only by taking 30 diazepam tablets.

【Examination】

Emaciation, listlessness, dull eyes, dark complexion, tearing eyes and runny nose, pale red tongue, thin white coating, deep weak pulse.

【Diagnosis】

Heroin withdrawal syndrome (due to yang deficiency with toxins deposited in the interior)

【Treatment Principles】

Restore yang, conduct toxins out.

【Treatment】

SJ 6 (*zhī gōu*)	DU 20 (*bǎi huì*)

An even method, with the needles retained for 50 minutes. Treated so he experienced a gentle and comfortable needling sensation. After five minutes his nose cleared up and he felt clear minded, the tearing also stopped. The needles were manipulated every 10 minutes by scratching the handle 9 times, which is a yang figure, with the meaning to lead to yang.

During the acupuncture treatment the patient felt comfortable, almost like being relaxed by smoking heroin. That night he did not need any medicine to fall asleep. At midnight he woke with the usual withdrawal symptoms of joint pain, irritability, tearing eyes and a runny nose. With the help of massage and 4 diazepam tablets he slept again with difficulty.

The second visit:

DU 20 (bǎi huì)	SJ 6 (zhī gōu)	LI 11 (qū chí)
LI 4 (hé gǔ)	LV 3 (tài chōng)	SP 6 (sān yīn jiāo)

The same technique was applied. After about 10 minutes the patient felt irritable and ached all over the body. The adjustment of the needle sensation and spiritual comfort calmed him down again. The needles were retained for two hours, during which time he slept briefly twice. Two hours later the dizziness and pain stopped, he felt hungry and clear minded.

This patient was treated a total of 10 times. He became energetic again and went back to his work.

【Note】

This is a syndrome of yang deficiency with the drug toxin deposited in the interior and qi and blood deficiency. The treatment should aim at restoring yang and driving the toxin out. Main points: SJ 6 (zhī gōu) is to regulate the san jiao and promote yang qi to drive the toxin out; DU 20 (bǎi huì) is to restore yang and reinforce qi. Acupuncture - moxibustion is an effective and simple way to help addicts cope with the withdrawal from heroin, and clear toxins from the body.

Summary

Withdrawal syndrome refers to the group of symptoms that appear when withdrawing from alcohol, tobacco or heroin. Acupuncture is an ideal therapy in treating addiction to various substances. Its advantage is not only that it can help patients withdraw, but also that it can help them to stay drug free. Although there have been many clinical and experimental studies, the selection of points and their functional mechanism need to be studied further.

MAIN REFERENCES

1. Wang Zuo-liang, Xu Yu-sheng, Lu Yan-yao rectifies. *Lu Shou-yan's Medical Records on Acupuncture*. Shanghai: Shanghai Scientific and Technical Publishers; 2008

2. Yang Yi-fang, et al. rectifies. *Selections from Yang Yong-xuan's Medical Records on Acupuncture*. Shanghai: Shanghai Scientific and Technical Publishers; 2002

3. Liu Bing-quan, Tang Yu-lan. *Selections from Yang Yong-xuan's Medical Records on Acupuncture*. Guangdong: Guangdong Scientific and Technical Publishers; 2002

4. Yang Jie-bin. *Selections from Yang Jie-bin's Clinical Experience*. Beijing: China Medico-Pharmaceutical Sciences and Technology Publishing House; 2001

5. Liu Guan-jun. *Selections from the Medical Records of Modern Acupuncture Therapy*. Beijing: The People's Medical Publishing House; 1985

INDEX BY POINT NAMES

T

W

X

Y

Z

INDEX BY *PIN YIN*

INDEX BY DISEASE NAMES

图书在版编目（CIP）数据

名家针灸医案解读（英文）/ 王宏才编著. —北京：人民
卫生出版社，2009.8
ISBN 978-7-117-11808-8

Ⅰ. 名… Ⅱ. 王… Ⅲ. 针灸疗法－医案－研究－中国－
英文 Ⅳ. R245

中国版本图书馆 CIP 数据核字（2009）第 055673 号

门户网：**www.pmph.com**	出版物查询、网上书店
卫人网：**www.hrhexam.com**	执业护士、执业医师、 卫生资格考试培训

名家针灸医案解读（英文）

编　　著：王宏才
出版发行：人民卫生出版社(中继线+8610-6761-6688）
地　　址：中国北京市丰台区方庄芳群园三区 3 号楼
邮　　编：100078
E - mail：pmph @ pmph.com
发　　行：pmphsales@gmail.com
购书热线：+8610-6769-1034（电话及传真）
开　　本：710×1000　1/16
版　　次：2009 年 8 月第 1 版　2009 年 8 月第 1 版第 1 次印刷
标准书号：ISBN 978-7-117-11808-8/R·11809

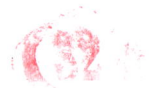

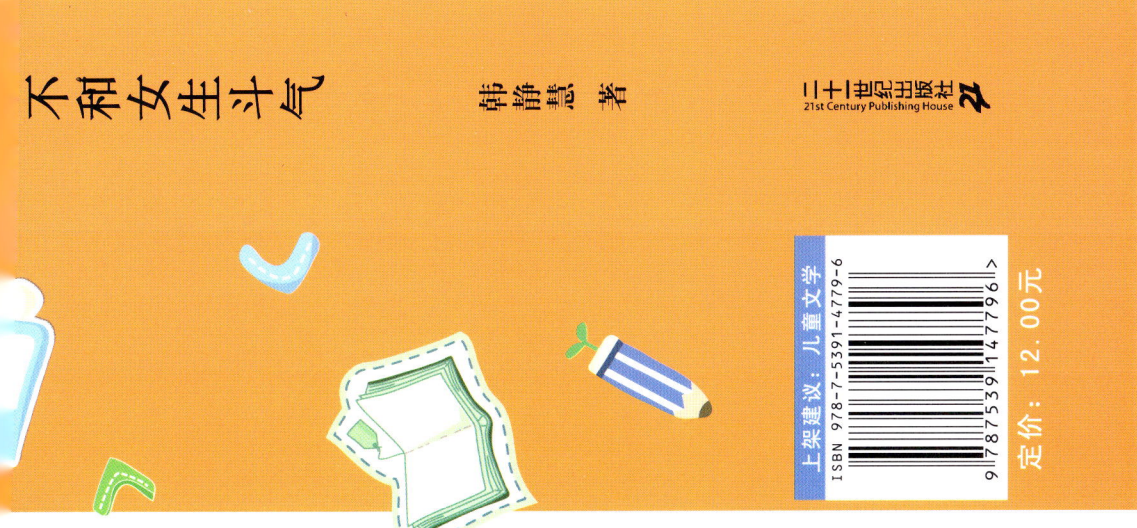

不和女生斗气

韩静慧 著

二十一世纪出版社
21st Century Publishing House

上架建议：儿童文学
ISBN 978-7-5391-4779-6
定价：12.00元

成长中的少年人，情感世界是丰富多彩的。作家韩静慧怀着热切的期望和真诚的心，以轻松活泼的笔调，写下了这青春的印记，生命的花朵。

著名作家、著名儿童文学评论家 **金波**

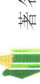《神秘女生》是作家韩静慧历时三年给孩子们打造出的一套集故事性、文学性、思想性、幽默性、人文性、知识性、教育性于一体的好作品，可谓是一套亲子阅读的精品之作。

著名作家、著名儿童文学评论家 **樊发稼**

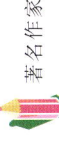当我读到米末、麦娜、夏林和桑琪等神秘而阳光的男生女生的故事时，我觉得他们有我童年的影子，而且这些形象所散发出的生命气息，他们的自信、诚实、智慧，快乐和单纯感染着我，让我体验到了童心世界所有的美好。

著名作家、著名儿童文学评论家 **谭旭东**

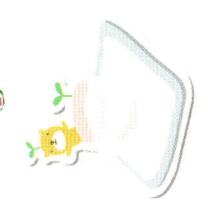